W9-DDM-372

The Care and Management
of the
Sick and Incompetent Physician

The Care and Management
of the
Sick and Incompetent Physician

By

ROBERT C. GREEN, JR., M.D.

Past President, Virginia State Board of Medicine

GEORGE J. CARROLL, M.D.

Secretary-Treasurer, Virginia State Board of Medicine

WILLIAM D. BUXTON, M.D.

Chairman, Psychiatric Advisory Committee
Virginia State Board of Medicine

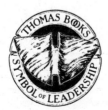

CHARLES C THOMAS • PUBLISHER
Springfield · Illinois · U.S.A.

Published and Distributed Throughout the World by

CHARLES C THOMAS • PUBLISHER

Bannerstone House

301-327 East Lawrence Avenue, Springfield, Illinois, U.S.A.

© *1978, by* CHARLES C THOMAS • PUBLISHER

ISBN 0-398-03727-2

Library of Congress Catalog Card Number: 77-21401

With THOMAS BOOKS *careful attention is given to all details of
manufacturing and design. It is the Publisher's desire to present books that
are satisfactory as to their physical qualities and artistic possibilities and
appropriate for their particular use.* THOMAS BOOKS *will be true to those
laws of quality that assure a good name and good will.*

Printed in the United States of America
R-1

Library of Congress Cataloging in Publication Data

Green, Robert C
    The care and management of the sick and
incompetent physician.

    Bibliography: p.
    Includes index.
    1. Physicians--Diseases and hygiene--United States.
2. Physicians--Mental health--United States.   3. Phy-
sicians--United States--Discipline.   4. Medical laws
and legislation--United States.   I. Carroll, George J.,
joint author.   II. Buxton, William D., joint author.
III. Title.   [DNLM: 1. Physicians--United States.
2. Clinical competence.   3. Ethics, Medical.   W21
G797c]
RA399.A3G77   610.69'52   77-21401
ISBN 0-398-03727-2

FOREWORD

AMONG the more altruistic of our colleagues are those physicians who voluntarily serve on statutory boards of medical licensure. They assume this onerous and often thankless obligation on behalf of the practitioners who live and practice within a given jurisdiction.

The practice of medicine presupposes adherence to an ethico-moral code. Every medical student on the occasion of his graduation has sworn to abide by the Oath of Hippocrates since the Golden Age of Pericles in the 4th century B.C. These lofty ideals have come to us, these twenty-odd centuries later, as a secular rite of passage. It has been the spirit of that oath as well as the social conscience of Socrates, a contemporary of Hippocrates, that has required that the profession of medicine, in the words of Robert Louis Stevenson, ". . . stand above the common herd." It is the duty of the several state medical boards to monitor adherence to these high standards of competence and ethical conduct.

David Hume, the Scottish moral philosopher, pointed out, over two hundred years ago, the logical gap between factual statements and moral judgments; or as it is put these days — between "is" and "ought." This is-ought dilemma is surely the central moral problem that besets the human condition.

A pivotal tenet of organized society holds that the warrant to compel an adult member to perform or to desist from performing an act, rests squarely on the benefit or harm that the action is likely to produce. This fundamental principle shapes the social structure of society. It is the basis of legal as well as moral order that governs conduct and regulates interpersonal relations. It legitimates rights as well as grants privileges. It confers license; by the same token it levies sanctions for transgressions.

In this regard, medicine occupies a unique position among the professions by virtue of its practitioners being granted an unusual privilege that vests in them the grave, societal responsibility of care and tending of the sick and disabled. Incidental to the discharge of these medical ministration, physicians have to be privy to the entire person of each of their patients. The tacit stipulations of the informal contract that governs such total access by physicians are the substance of the Hippocratic tradition. The patient is expected to fulfill his part of this contractual relationship by trusting his physician and therefore complying with the physician's instructions. There are inferential historical data that hold that from time to time these bilateral requirements have been more honored in the breach than in their compliance.

The reasons for the noncompliance are obvious. Physicians are human and consequently fallible, subject to the same vagaries and defections as other men and women. Patients as humans too are even more prone to human frailties being sick and thus susceptible to suggestion and exploitation. *Autre temps, autre moeurs,* human rights and ethico-moral obligations have become politicized these days. As such they are now ripe subjects for litigation. Then too, these days few values enjoy the status or the permanence of the traditional eternal verities. Cultural evolution continually changes our perspectives and consequently our perceptions. No longer is "truth" ascertained by ordeals of water or fire. Technology since the Industrial Revolution has innovated values both by creating previously unobtainable options as well as by changing the relative costs of existing options.

There seems to be a growing consensus that the laissez-faire attitude of earlier times that upheld the autonomous, self-regulating character of professional medical organizations is viewed as potentially exploitive. This belief has been restated by a related 1975 Supreme Court decision which held that regulations creating state boards of control are ". . . at the core of the state's power to protect the public." In recent times in support of this thesis, there has been a proliferation of federal, state and local regulatory bodies. In response, various medical groups, in the belief that this encroachment must be forestalled, have undertaken moves to assure the public of adequate safeguards: periodic examinations are given to attest the competence of their members. Such increasing emphasis of quality control is reflected in the *pro bono publico* movement; manifestly these watch-dog groups are designed with the expressed conviction that there may be laxity on the part of public institutions in the discharge of their fiduciary responsibility and the citizenry has an inalienable right-to-know.

These elements constitute the psychosocial and chronological contexts which have to be seen and understood as motivating factors in Doctors Green, Carroll, and Buxton's undertaking the survey of "The Care and Management of the Sick and Incompetent Physician."

The monograph is a compilation of information that, as officers of the Virginia State Board of Medicine, the authors have learned to define the many problems of physicians whose incompetence causes them to come within the purview of the board's official concern.

Their stated purpose is twofold. Admitting the deficiencies in the available data they provide a demographic account of the stewardship of the Virginia State Board of Medicine. Incidental to this parochial reflection on the types and prevalence of problems of Virginia physicians, the survey is interlarded with the related experience of others. The second purpose is a laudable therapeutic effort to respond in a positive fashion to the biblical admonition: physician, heal thyself. With the establishment of a Psychiatric Advisory Committee, the Virginia physicians practice what they preach. The Psychiatric Advisory Committee is composed of a neutral, professional competent group formed to assist the board in its deliberations.

The book is an annotated elaboration of a widespreading movement on the part of many state medical societies. It is a welcome extension of the work of the Council on Mental Health of the American Medical Association. Further, it provides preliminary data on the knowledge of etiology and prevalence of these morbid conditions in a physician population.

HOWARD P. ROME, M. D.
Professor of Psychiatry (Emeritus)
Mayo Graduate School of Medicine
Past Chairman of the Council on
      Mental Health, American Medical
      Association

PREFACE

MANAGEMENT of physicians whose competence is compromised by mental or physical illness, alcoholism, drug addiction, lack of diligence in keeping abreast of current practices, or other factors traditionally has been considered the responsibility of the medical profession itself. A trusting society has tended to assume that the profession would conscientiously regulate its own members. Increasingly, however, it has become evident that existing disciplinary mechanisms have been poorly utilized and that hospital staffs and state licensing agencies have evinced little enthusiasm for effective action against violators of even the most basic professional and ethical standards.

The public, government officials, and leading members of the profession are now showing increasing concern in the matter of physician competence and deviant behavior and are demanding prompt and effective action by medical disciplinary bodies.

Management of the sick and/or incompetent physician is not simple. In fact, even identifying these physicians often represents a problem for those responsible for disciplinary action. At the same time, an absence of effective and realistic laws and guidance at all levels further limits a resolution of the problem.

The purpose of this monograph is to present an in-depth study of the sick, incompetent, or unethical physician. Utilizing the experience of the Virginia State Board of Medicine and that of others, we try to identify various types of mental illness among physicians and to provide guidelines for recognizing such illness. In addition, we will outline mechanisms at both the state and local levels for adequately handling these problems. The management and rehabilitation of those physicians so unfortunate as to become professionally incompetent because of drugs, alcohol, mental illness, senility, or physical

ix

disability will also be discussed.

It is our hope that the bringing together of extensive information concerning sick and/or incompetent physicians will provide an impetus to better management of a growing problem within the medical profession and thereby provide the public with safeguards and protection which have not existed in the past.

ACKNOWLEDGMENTS

THE authors are indebted to Walter L. Penn, III, former Assistant Attorney General of the State of Virginia, for his authorship of Chapter 7 on "Legal Rights of the Sick or Incompetent Physician." We also wish to give recognition to the other members of the Virginia State Board of Medicine and to the members of the Psychiatric Advisory Committee for their support and encouragement of this work. However, the opinions expressed in this book are the responsibility of the authors and are not necessarily those of the Board.

The authors wish to thank F. Juanita Mayo, Executive Secretary, Peggy Neville and Nancy Spain, secretaries, for their help in assembling our data, and Sylvia S. Covet for her patient and careful editing of the manuscript.

R.C.G.
G.J.C.
W.D.B.

CONTENTS

The Care and Management
of the
Sick and Incompetent Physician

Chapter 1

THE DEMAND FOR
PROFESSIONAL DISCIPLINE

SINCE the end of World War II, a change has
gradually evolved in the attitude of the public toward the medical profession. During the preceding century, the public's attitude had been one of reverence. In many instances the
relationship between the patient and his physician was more
"sacred" than his relationship with his clergyman.

The attitudinal change has been due in part to the explosive
growth of medical knowledge during the twentieth century.
With the advent of the sulfonamides in the 1940s, an even more
rapid growth in medical knowledge occurred. Unfortunately,
this "explosion" of scientific knowledge has brought with it
many new problems for the practicing physician.

One major problem is the increasing pressure on the individual physician to keep abreast of rapidly changing patterns
of health care delivery. These pressures are part of the reason
for ever-increasing numbers of problems among physicians.
Another factor is the overall increase in the number of doctors.
Applications to medical schools each year number in the
hundreds of thousands. This increase in applications results in
many problems in the selection process which, in turn, leads to
an increase in the number of "problem physicians."

Studies conducted as long ago as the 1930s illustrated the
potential for problems in medical school classes. One 1937
study showed that "slightly more than 46 percent of senior
students in a representative medical school suffer from neurotic
handicaps of a major character."[1] Dowling,[2] in 1955, revealed
that 10,000 doctors surveyed, 0.5 percent replied affirmatively
regarding the presence of a psychiatric disorder. In this same
survey, two different medical school classes reported an incidence of 6.5 and 13 percent respectively of each class who had

been or were currently under the care of a psychiatrist.

The physician of the mid-1970s has had to make some major adjustments to changes in the practice of medicine. For example, although government controls on the medical profession are not new — serious efforts in this direction began in the 1940s — they have increased tremendously in recent years. As a result, the physician is faced with ever-increasing surveillance of his practice.

Two trends which have had a profound effect on physician-patient relationships and on the incidence of problem physicians are apparent in the latter half of the twentieth century. First is the increase in specialization and subspecialization, and second is a major move toward group practice.

With group practice, clinics, and health maintenance organizations (HMOs), the patient does not develop the same kind of relationship that he may have had with an individual physician practicing alone. The number of specialties and subspecialties often bewilders patients and decreases their sense of trust in the profession. This results in a general change of attitude toward all physicians — often to one of impatience, frustration, or hostility. No doubt this has contributed to the increase in malpractice suits that has plagued the profession in recent years.

Physicians involved in medical licensure and disciplinary procedures are aware that these conditions often lead to serious problems for individual physicians. There is a continuing search for optimum ways to handle problem physicians. The goal is rehabilitation when possible, but effective and fair disciplinary action when necessary. The Virginia State Board of Medicine strongly believes that a large percentage of physicians who come under its scrutiny can be salvaged and returned to active practice and that in only a small percentage of cases will permanent disciplinary action be necessary.

Historically, the medical profession has accepted the responsibility of disciplining its own; society, intimidated by the complexities of medical practice, has willingly allowed the profession to assume this responsibility. Unfortunately, past self-disciplinary efforts have been inadequate, due largely to the traditional fraternal bonds that exist in the profession and to an unwillingness to acknowledge that the incompetent or deviant physician is not a rare phenomenon. Consequently, until recent years, significant disciplinary action has been a rare occurrence, except in the most extreme cases. In short, physicians have been loath to act as their brothers' keepers.

As the government has increased its intrusion into all aspects of medical practice — hospitals, laboratories, private examining rooms, and pharmacies — and as the public has become embued with "consumerism," the medical profession suddenly has "more keepers than physicians."[3]

The press is full of reports of fraud, abuse, and the more sensational malpractice suits. Congress is considering legislation to strengthen the capability of the federal government to detect, prosecute, and punish fraudulent activities under the Medicaid and Medicare programs.[4] In addition, major Medicare and Medicaid reimbursement reform legislation is pending, as is a bill to stringently regulate clinical laboratories. Various plans for national health insurance are under consideration which, if enacted, will place the government right in the center of the practice of medicine. The medical profession *must* take cognizance of this activity and *must* begin to discipline its own members more effectively. Physicians themselves are more qualified for this task than any other group, but if they do not do it, others will, with less effectiveness and less compassion.

In 1958, the American Medical Association (AMA) formally acknowledged the problem of self-discipline within the profession by establishing the first Medical Disciplinary Committee. The committee's purpose was to provide effective factual information and to assess accurately the status of medical discipline. The result of that study, published in 1961, was a devastating conclusion that there was "apathy, substantial ignorance, and a lack of a sense of individual responsibility by physicians as a whole toward discipline in organized medicine."[5] Following this statement, thirty specific recommendations were made by the Medical Disciplinary Committee in its report to the AMA Board of Trustees. For example, medical schools were urged to develop courses in ethics and socioeconomic principles; state licensing boards were told to consider seriously the advisability and necessity of making discipline their primary responsibility; state medical associations were urged to utilize grievance committees to initiate action against offenders; and the AMA was suggested as the repository and clearinghouse of all major disciplinary actions taken by state boards.

Reinforcing this initial AMA effort to stimulate the medical profession to clean house was a 1965 landmark legal decision in *Darling vs Charleston Memorial Community Hospital.*[6] Essentially, this decision stated that a hospital administration can be held responsible for the competence of staff members. In the same year, Medicare and Medicaid legislation was passed, and with the growing possibility of national health insurance, there were increasing signs that eligibility for federal remuneration would be related to documentation of physician competence. Since these landmark actions by the AMA, the courts, and the Congress, there has been a rising demand both within and outside the medical profession for greater accountability by organized medicine for the impaired and incompetent physician.

Coupled with this demand has been a growing realization that recognition and motivation for reform were needed just as much as or more than effective legal and procedural guidelines. Thus, in 1967, the Federation of State Licensing Boards,[7] alarmed by the increasing numbers of physicians addicted to alcohol and drugs, presented a resolution to the AMA House of Delegates imploring recognition of this problem. These pioneering efforts met with limited concern and only perfunctory attention. However, they impelled much delayed recognition of these occupational hazards afflicting physicians and, in particular, of drug addiction and the high incidence of alcoholism, and the incompetence associated with these abuses.

It has generally been recognized that, for many years, the vagaries and limitations of state laws regulating medical practice were limiting factors in effectively disciplining incompetent and deviant physicians. Without strong pressures and guidance from leaders of the medical profession, little was done to correct this weakness in disciplinary procedures and laws until 1969. In that year, the Florida State Board of Medicine, in conjunction with the state legislature, proposed and secured passage of a landmark legislative bill commonly referred to as the "Sick Doctor Statute."[8] This act replaced the previous grounds for medical discipline, which had been predicated on the commission by a physician of one or more enumerated items of misconduct, which varied from state to state and required proof of fault. The new Florida Sick Doctor Statute provided jurisdiction over physicians who were unable to practice medicine with reasonable skill and safety because of any medical or emotional cause.

This legislative model gave the medical profession an effective method of disciplining sick and incompetent practitioners at both the state and local levels. Florida's legislative example also exerted further pressure on the medical profession to enforce discipline among its ranks.

Accompanying the passage of Medicare and Medicaid legislation has been an increasing demand for the profession to ensure that all physicians maintain their clinical competence. Concurrently, there has been a general dissatisfaction with the concept of licensure for life, the prevailing custom in all states as a result of generally automatic licensure renewal.

Responding to these events and a leadership effort by Doctor Robert Derbyshire, former president of the State Federation of Medical Boards, New Mexico passed a bill in 1971 requiring 150 hours of continuing education every three years, thereby establishing the first mandatory requirement toward continuing clinical competence. Since that time, at least eighteen other state legislatures have passed similar bills in an effort to provide better medical care and to show the public that the medical profession is attempting to maintain a strong disciplinary posture. In addition, many state medical societies now require proof of continuing education for membership.

Further pressures to exercise discipline and ensure competence came from federal legislation enacted in 1972 to establish Professional Standards Review Organizations (PSROs). In the same year, the AMA Council on Mental Health, in an attempt to define the profession's responsibility toward deviant practitioners, stated that physicians have an "ethical responsibility to take cognizance of a colleague's inability to practice medicine adequately by reason of physical or mental illness, including alcoholism and drug dependence."[9] The Council further proceeded to outline the progressive steps that a concerned physician should follow. Until then, there had been no precise official statement that each individual physician has a responsibility to his profession and his colleagues and is indeed "his brother's keeper."

Despite increasing pressure for disciplinary reform over the past decade, progress has been slow. A widely quoted survey of state medical boards covering a period of over twenty years found that only a very few licenses had been revoked each year. This kind of record reflects continued apathy on the part of members of the medical profession and spurs the demand for disciplinary reform from many directions. The professional literature is also replete with criticism.[10-12] This emphasis on the need for action has now affected other professional groups, and many national professional societies in all fields are experiencing similar pressures.

Reflecting these pressures for disciplinary reform, in 1975 the AMA sponsored a national conference aptly titled, "The Disabled Doctor — Challenge to the Profession."[13] Here, for the first time, leaders in the field comprehensively reviewed the problems of impaired and incompetent physicians and the proper procedures for local and state authorities to follow. This conference was the first of a series to produce increasing grass-roots recognition and knowledge of the need for discipline in the medical profession. The second conference, sponsored by the AMA Department of Mental Health and the Medical Association of Georgia, was held in Atlanta in early February 1977 and was called, "The Impaired Physician: Answering the Challenge." A summary report of the conference will be published by the AMA.

There is an ever-increasing public sophistication and knowledge about medical problems, disease processes, and treatment. As the public's medical expectations have grown, so has the need for accountability on the part of the profession. Widespread patient dissatisfaction with the quality of health care received has been mirrored by extensive publicity[14, 15] as well as by legislative efforts.

All of these forces, both within and without the profession, have been effective; organized medicine is at last doing something about the incompetent and deviant physician.

State licensing boards have proved to be effective instruments for disciplinary action. While hospital boards and medical societies can censure and reprimand, they do not offer protection to patients. The sole effective method of curtailing a physician's practice is by revoking his license, a view supported by Doctor John H. Budd, 1976 president-elect of the AMA. In an interview, Budd said, "You see, doctors are not licensed by the AMA or by medical societies. Doctors are licensed by medical practice boards. The biggest problem in disciplining doctors is to get the support of the state licensing boards."

It is vital that the deviant, incompetent, or "sick" doctor be reported and disciplined. If such a physician is allowed to continue to practice, he himself, his patients, and the entire medical profession are all losers. The doctor's torment is prolonged, his patients' lives are endangered, and the profession's standards are lowered. The need for medical discipline is great. The public demands it, the government demands it, and the medical profession *must* demand it.

REFERENCES

1. Strecker, E. A., Appel, K. E., Palmer, H. D., and Braceland, F. J.: Psychiatric studies in medical education. II. Neurotic trends in senior medical students. *Am J Psychiatry, 93*:1197-1229, 1937.
2. Dowling, H. F.: Physician, heal thyself. *GP, 11*:69-73, 1955.
3. Crawshaw, R. S.: Who is my brother's keeper? *Federation Bull, 58*:364-372, 1971.
4. Medicare-Medicaid Anti-Fraud and Abuse Amendments. H. R. 3, S. 143, Ninety-fifth Congress, First Session, January 4, 1977 and January 11, 1977.
5. Report of AMA Medical Disciplinary Committee to Board of Trustees, 67-73, June 1961.
6. Darling vs Charleston Community Memorial Hospital, 50 Ill. App. 2d 253, 200 N.E. 2d 149 (4th Cir., 1964); *Aff'd* 33 Ill. 2d 326, 211 N.E. 2d

253 (1965), *cert. denied,* 383 U.S. 946 (1966).

7. Casterline, R. L.: Editorial. *Federation Bull, 60*:29-30, 1973.

8. (a) Sec 2, 69-205, LAWS OF FLORIDA; (b) FLORIDA STATUTE 458-1201(1)(N).

9. AMA Council on Mental Health: The sick physician; impairment by psychiatric disorders, including alcoholism and drug dependence. *JAMA 223*:684-687, 1973.

10. Derbyshire, R. C.: Medical ethics and discipline. *JAMA, 228*:59-62, 1974.

11. Warren, D. G.: Discipline of physicians. *J Leg Med,* 2:23-26, 1974.

12. Kilpatrick, J. J.: The Medicaid Medicare ripoffs — Where is the medical profession? *Winchester Evening Star,* 4, Tues., Aug. 17, 1976.

13. Steindler, E. M.: *The Impaired Physician: An Interpretive Summary of the AMA Conference on "The Disabled Doctor: Challenge to the Profession."* AMA Department of Mental Health, 1-54, April 11-12, 1975.

14. Lublin, J. S.: Do doctors need a check-up? *Wall Street Journal,* Feb. 25, 1974.

15. Rensberger, B.: Unfit doctors; Incompetent surgery; Thousand a year killed by faulty prescriptions; Few doctors ever report colleagues' incompetence; How educated patients get proper care. The New York Times, Jan. 26-30, 1976.

Chapter 2

MAINTAINING PROFESSIONAL COMPETENCE

AMONG the more difficult problems that now confront members of the medical profession is continuing professional competence. Aside from an estimated 5 percent of mentally ill, drug-addicted, and alcoholic physicians, there remains approximately 95 percent of the medical profession who were presumed competent at the onset of their careers. These physicians are expected to provide a high standard of medical care, according to the latest scientifically accepted diagnostic and therapeutic procedures. The problem is how to assure the public this high level of performance throughout the professional lifetime of a practicing physician.

Traditionally, the public has delegated the responsibility for maintaining physician competence to the profession itself, through the legislation of state medical practice acts, and has given the authority for licensing to the state medical boards. Society has allowed the profession to be largely self-governed in the belief that only members of the medical profession have the knowledge and expertise necessary to effectively control its own members. Now, however, the public is questioning how well the medical profession has met this trust. Increasing medical sophistication on the part of the public and more media coverage of medical procedures and other aspects of health care have brought increased pressure on the profession to insure the competence of its members and to make this effort visible. With growing frequency, pressures and criticisms have been directed toward state medical boards, since they are the legally constituted bodies within each state that are directly responsible to the public for insuring professional competence.

Until recent years, state medical boards were primarily concerned with demonstrating a physician's competence only at his completion of medical school, with little thought given to his competence in the later years of practice. When licensing boards did recognize the problem of clinical incompetence after the initial licensing, the problem was usually associated with such deviant behavior as drug addiction, chronic alcoholism, or mental illness.

There have been many reasons for this rather narrow attention to medical competence. In the past, it was assumed that a license to practice medicine entitled a physician to practice a lifetime, provided that there was no evidence of gross incompetence associated with either addiction or severe emotional problems. It was loosely assumed that physicians would be self-motivated to continue their medical education in a meaningful and productive fashion throughout the duration of their clinical practice; hence physicians would remain continuously competent. The "right" of physicians to practice for life has now come under increasing criticism because of the current generally accepted concept that those who do not remain lifelong students face professional obsolescence within five to ten years after receiving their medical degrees. It has also been belatedly recognized that there is no assurance that all physicians are sufficiently motivated intellectually to commit themselves to the academic effort necessary to avoid professional deterioration.

The American Medical Association, state and local medical societies, teaching centers, and the specialty societies have traditionally provided educational programs and courses designed to meet the needs of practicing physicians. Unfortunately, the caliber, availability, and, particularly, the relevance of such courses have frequently been questioned. In addition, the concept of continuing education as it relates to clinical competence has come under extensive scrutiny. There are skeptics who challenge the effectiveness of these traditional educational formats to change and modify medical performance at the practicing level.

In 1969, an AMA report[1] on continuing competence of physicians acknowledged the need to provide incentives for physicians to maintain their clinical competence. This was one of the first official, although indirect, admissions that a problem did exist in regard to maintaining proficiency in clinical practice. In the years following this declaration, the AMA has encouraged continuing education through its Physician Recognition Award Program and has fostered the use of the educational requirements covered by the program for membership privileges in state medical societies and other professional associations. However, the AMA has limited its motivational stimulus to an entirely voluntary effort. In effect, the AMA has acknowledged the problem of motivating physicians to keep abreast of new information and thus practice competent medicine. At the same time, however, the AMA has continued to support the "right" to practice undeterred for life once an initial state license has been granted. It should be noted that with the increasing emphasis on continuing medical education, a physician who is markedly deficient in his acquisition of current information, in some instances, may lose his membership in a general medical or specialty society. Nevertheless, the physician is still legally allowed to practice medicine. It is indeed strange that acknowledgment of the importance of continuing education extends to expulsion of a physician from a professional organization but does not protect the patient whom he treats.

What problems do most physicians face in keeping their professional skills current? Motivation is, of course, one of the most basic concerns. After completing residency training, physicians are usually enthusiastic about and dedicated to the academic world to which they have been exposed for so many years. However, on entering the "real world" of medical practice, much can and often does happen over the years to erode the motivation of even the most conscientious physician.

Many physicians become physically or geographically isolated from their peers and from the mainstream of medical innovation and advancement. With the passage of time, their core of medical knowledge imperceptibly shrinks, and there is an accompanying decreased level of performance which the physician himself often does not notice. Even those who remain motivated toward excellence but are in an isolated situation find it difficult to maintain a high level of medical performance. Isolated physicians who have been brought to the attention of the Virginia State Board of Medicine for minor infractions have repeatedly been found to have given only cursory attention to maintaining their competence. Seldom have these physicians undertaken even the most basic forms of continuing education. One need only contemplate the frequency of this type of physician isolation in order to estimate the extent of the problem.

Every successful physician finds that as his practice load increases, his available time becomes increasingly committed, with little time left for outside activities. As a result, however strong his motivation, less and less time may be devoted to maintaining an initial high level of clinical competence. As the average physician reaches middle age and achieves financial security, he may become involved in medical politics, hospital committee work, civic activities, and, sometimes, outside financial commitments, often leaving little time for family life, recreation, or other pursuits. Such factors gradually reduce both motivation and time for continuing medical education.

Finally, increasing age, with the accompanying gradual diminution of physical and mental vigor, further erodes motivation to maintain competence. It has often been said that the aging physician is seldom a threat to his patients because he gradually limits himself to the simpler clinical problems and avoids the more complex and intricate medical challenges. It is small comfort to his patients that the decision to limit his work depends on the aging physician's own insight and that if his self-evaluation is faulty, it is the patient not the physician who suffers the consequences.

To a limited degree, the medical profession, the public, and third-party payers have recognized the problems of maintaining professional competence. All three groups have made increasing demands for reassurance that the profession is handling this matter in a responsible manner.

Despite all the usurpations of motivation that may occur, many physicians do manage to devote a significant amount of time to maintaining their clinical skills. In any case, the time is past when a physician's knowledge and performance were automatically accepted and never questioned.

Various approaches have been devised to meet the challenge of assuring competence. In 1969, the AMA instituted its Physician Recognition Award Program, which requires 150 hours of specified types of continuing education every three years, with the requisite that 60 of these hours have approved sponsors. Physicians who follow this plan are awarded a certificate of completion of the program. However, no documentation of attendance or evaluation of participation is required before bestowal of the certificate. Nevertheless, the program has provided a quantitative measurement of the effort put forth by physicians who have been attempting to maintain professional competence. This has provided a measurement that the public can readily understand. How effective such hours are in changing and upgrading clinical performance is not as clearly defined.

In 1972, Medicare and Medicaid regulations were amended to create what was intended to be a more effective mechanism of providing adequate quality and cost control. The new law made it possible for groups of physicians in geographic areas designated by the federal government to contract with the Department of Health, Education, and Welfare (HEW) to establish Professional Standards Review Organizations. These PSRO groups were charged with the responsibility of establishing minimum standards of hospital care and of monitoring the quality and cost of services provided under Medicare and Medicaid. While PSROs have no direct control over physicians, by establishing standards they indirectly encourage an upgrading of quality, although skeptics argue that such standards are set at the lowest common denominator. Unfortunately, inadequate federal funding and a lack of enthusiasm on the part of the medical profession have made this program doubtfully effective in maintaining professional competence.

Peer review has been one of the most successful methods for evaluating physician performance. This has been vigorously advocated by the Joint Commission on Hospital Accreditation and has been effective primarily in large, highly structured hospitals. For institutions of a hundred beds or less, the program's effectiveness is limited because the very intimacy of professional relationships in small institutions makes effective peer review difficult, if not impossible. Further, the time required to conduct effective peer review, with all its ramifications, is a limiting factor.

In an attempt to resolve the problem of professional obsolescence, specialty boards began voluntary recertification programs for their diplomates, based on written examinations. In 1973, the American Board of Medical Specialties recommended to all member boards that voluntary periodic recertification of medical specialists become an integral part of all national medical specialty certification programs, and that a deadline be established when voluntary periodic recertification of medical specialists would become a standard policy. Since this policy-making declaration, there have been further pressures to *require* periodic reexamination for maintaining specialty certification.

There have, of course, been numerous objections to the reexamination concept. Concern has been expressed as to whether the results of any challenge examination can directly relate to a level of performance in practice and, indeed, whether such examinations can define the relevant dimensions of clinical competence in any specialty. Further, it has been felt that assessment by actual performance is the preferred and only meaningful approach to evaluating the abilities of practicing physicians. Unfortunately, techniques for this type of evaluation of a physician's performance are not now and may never be available.

Even if voluntary or mandatory recertifying examinations for the specialties become a part of the American medical scene, this approach still fails to remove the educationally incompetent physician from the practice of medicine. Loss of certification may produce limitation of privileges in some cases, but for the most part it probably will have little effect on a physician's exposure to patients. Certainly it will have no effect on his office practice. It should also be noted that, at present, only approximately half of all physicians practicing in the United States are certified.

Since its founding in 1949, the American Academy of Family Physicians has required a specific number of hours of continuing education as a condition for membership. In 1970, the Oregon State Medical Association became the first state medical society to require participation in continuing education programs as a condition for membership. Since then, at least a dozen other state societies have adopted this requirement. Unfortunately, noncompliance results only in loss of membership in the state society, with virtually no accompanying limitation of practice privileges. It must be recognized, too, that many physicians do not belong to state medical societies, and such mandatory requirements for continuing membership do not affect this nonmember group.

If the ultimate responsibility for maintaining competence is to remain totally with the profession, there must be some way to encompass the entire field of medicine in an article of faith that is apparent to the public and readily understood. Such a system must include all of the previously discussed methods of insuring competence and also be backed by enforcement authority. At present the only proposal that adequately addresses itself to the maintenance of competence is mandatory continuing education for relicensure. Such a program would establish minimal annual educational requirements through the various specialty groups and state medical societies, with the authority for compliance vested in the state boards of medicine. This is the only way to insure that every practicing physician will at least be exposed to a significant number of hours of continuing education. Only through such programs can the medical profession restore public confidence in its determination to see that every practicing physician remains professionally competent. Annual educational requirements for relicensure were first adopted by the State of New Mexico; since then, the idea has been implemented by many other states. States that have instituted this type of program have reported that the number and caliber of continuing education courses available to physicians have improved tremendously and that attendance has increased appreciably at state medical society meetings and programs.

Critics of mandatory continuing education for relicensure

argue that such a system will impose undue hardships on rural physicians who do not have ready access to educational programs or that they are unable to leave their practice to attend the programs. This is true, of course, but so many methods of obtaining acceptable credit hours are now available that this problem is probably more imaginary than real. Another question might also be asked, "Is an out-of-date, obsolescent physician essential to any community?"

Additional criticism of the mandatory approach points out that many approved methods of continuing education lack confirmatory controls and that physicians could easily make false reports of their educational activities without fear of discovery. Although this is true in some cases, we doubt very much that it would be a significant factor. Most states require a specific number of credit hours of AMA-accredited and formal courses at which a record of attendance is signed and certificates of course completion are given.

Are the existing methods of insuring competence sufficient? Will peer review and PSROs really upgrade the quality of medical care? Will relicensure requiring evidence of continuing medical education really change patterns of practice? In short, the basic question is whether continuing education really changes anything for the better.

The answer to all of these questions cannot be a resounding "yes," supported by sophisticated studies. There is, in fact, little basic information available on learning and behavior change at clinical practice levels, and no single procedure intended to evaluate performance as distinguished from knowledge has gained acceptance. To our dismay, we have been unable to find any definition of competence in clinical practice that we can follow. An exception may be the definition proposed by Doctor R. C. Derbyshire,* who stated that competence is "practicing good medicine by modern methods." The vagueness of this definition is apparent when one tries to define "good" or "modern" in this context.

Regrettably, even the most respected centers of medical edu-

---

*Doctor Derbyshire is Secretary-treasurer, New Mexico State Board of Medical Examiners and Past President, Federation of State Medical Boards.

cation offer little guidance in defining effective learning methods. Many of these institutions continue to use teaching formats developed as many as twenty years ago, and there are virtually no firm data on the correlation of the results of these programs and satisfactory clinical performance. Consequently, it is not surprising that the field of continuing education and the maintenance of physician competence are in such turmoil.

We are left then with unanswered questions: How can competence be defined? How can competence be assessed and assured? Final answers to these questions are so far not available, but until they are forthcoming, the profession must continue with multiple approaches and methods. Above all, the profession must convincingly reassure the public that maintaining clinical competence among physicians is foremost in its concern, and that it is an area in which definitive action is being taken and continuously reviewed.

REFERENCES

1. Report. What should the profession do about the incompetent physician? *JAMA, 194*:119-122, 1969.

Chapter 3

THE DRUG-ADDICTED PHYSICIAN

THE incidence of drug addiction among physicians is generally conceded to be high, an estimated ratio of 1:100 physicians as compared to 1:3000 in the general population.[1] In our opinion, this estimate is probably low and represents only a fraction of all physician addicts. Indeed, we consider drug addiction an occupational hazard for physicians. Despite this apparent high incidence of addiction, few studies have been published on any sizable number of cases, and available studies report only limited and fragmented aspects of the problem.

Our experience with drug-addicted physicians has been unique in that there has been an opportunity to follow the progress or failure of many addicted physicians for many years. From this disturbing and often heart-breaking experience, the Virginia State Board of Medicine has developed its own system of recognition, management, and rehabilitation of physician addicts.

This experience in Virginia with forty-six addicted physicians has been summarized,[2] but the study reflects only those cases in which significant data were collected.* Many of the physicians reported to us as addicted disappeared from follow-up and did not seek to renew their licenses or, in a few cases, committed suicide. In addition, many who were identified at the local level and confronted by their peers left the state to practice in a more permissive environment or convinced their colleagues that they had conquered the habit. Undoubtedly, many of these physicians are still addicted and have yet to be rediscovered.

Sources of reports on physician addicts are of interest. As

---

*This study contains case reports extending from 1949 through the first quarter of 1974. The additional eighteen cases noted in Table 9-III (1974-1976) are not included, as the data were not available when the initial study was reported.

would be expected, state and federal narcotics inspectors have
far outnumbered other sources (Table 3-I), since sooner or later
addicted physicians develop prescribing patterns that are obvious signs of personal drug abuse.

TABLE 3-I

SOURCE OF INITIAL REPORT OF ADDICTED PHYSICIANS

State Pharmacy Investigator	21
Federal Narcotics Investigator	5
Institutions	10
Individuals	5
Patient	2
Other State Boards	2
Medical Society of Va.	1
	Total 46

It has been our policy to establish a very close working relationship with the Virginia State Board of Pharmacy, with the
understanding that bizarre and inappropriate drug-prescribing
habits as well as apparent self-prescribing of addictive drugs
would be reported to the Virginia State Board of Medicine.
Such reports automatically lead to an investigation and an
initial informal hearing. As a result of more pharmacy inspec-
tions and the cooperation of the State Board of Pharmacy, the
incidence of drug abuse reported has increased in the past several years.

Still of great concern, however, is the limited number of
physician addicts reported by their peers or their medical societies. It seems strange that an addiction which so often pro-
duces deterioration of judgment and abdication of responsibility, as well as erratic behavior, can remain undetected by
colleagues and only ultimately be discovered by state pharmacy
inspectors. One can only deduce that a major proportion of

physicians who may be aware of the problem tend to avoid it entirely, or are unable to recognize the typically deviant behavior patterns of addiction, or are indifferent to the detrimental impact physician addicts inevitably have on the profession.

In all fairness, it must be acknowledged that the drug-addicted physician and his characteristic patterns are not so common as to arouse the suspicion of every physician observer. Certainly, in the early stages of addiction and at the start of personality deterioration, only suspicions can be raised. It is also important to note that the principal, and often only, similarity between physician addicts and street addicts is the common bond of drug dependence (Table 3-II).

Our study shows that the usual physician reported for addiction is a general practitioner or an internist who has been in practice approximately eighteen years (Table 3-III). His median age is forty-five years at the time of reporting (Table 3-IV). As a rule he has been addicted only a year before manifestations of his addiction become conspicuous. However, it should not be assumed that long-term addiction is impossible without detection; in some of our cases the physicians were addicted as long as ten, sixteen, and even eighteen years before discovery (Table 3-V). Since it is quite possible for some addicted physicians to escape detection for many years, it is disturbing to contemplate the number of these physicians practicing on an unsuspecting public and clever enough to avoid detection.

Other characteristics of the addicted physician indicate that he is usually suffering from a moderately severe, progressive personality disorder. In our study, depression — either as pure depression or as manic depression — was the most frequent underlying psychiatric disturbance in those cases where a reliable psychiatric evaluation was available. Although depression was the most frequent personality disorder associated with addiction, additional patterns of abnormal behavior were also noted (Table 3-VI). From this study, we developed a composite profile of the typical physician addict reported to the board (Table 3-VII).

Other studies concerning the psychiatric background of drug-addicted physicians are limited. Winick,[3] using prospec-

TABLE 3-II

COMPARISON OF PHYSICIAN AND STREET ADDICT

(1) Begins using drugs about the age that street addict "burns out."

(1) Usually begins drug use in adolescence.

(2) Typically uses meperidine in pure form.

(2) Typically uses heroin in diluted form.

(3) Seldom overdoses.

(3) Frequently overdoses.

(4) Detoxification often difficult.

(4) Detoxification less difficult.

(5) Usually discovered accidentally following a routine check by a pharmacy inspector.

(5) Usually arrested during purchase of drugs, with drugs in possession or during a criminal act.

(6) Almost never associates with other physician addicts.

(6) Usually associates with other addicts.

(7) No insight into his drug use.

(7) Has a wry insight into drug use.

(8) Never introduced to drugs by his contemporaries.

(8) Frequently introduced to drugs by contemporaries.

(9) Prognosis for cure — good.

(9) Prognosis for cure — poor.

(10) Usually married.

(10) Usually unmarried.

(11) Usually not a member of minority group.

(11) Usually member of a minority group.

TABLE 3-III

YEARS IN MEDICAL PRACTICE
PRIOR TO INITIAL REPORT OF DRUG ADDICTION

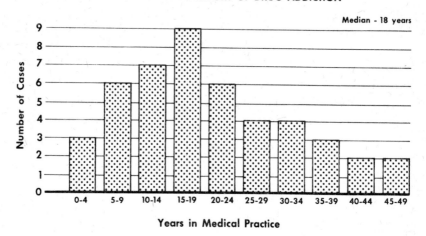

Median - 18 years

Years in Medical Practice

TABLE 3-IV

PHYSICIAN AGE AT TIME OF INITIAL REPORT OF DRUG ADDICTION

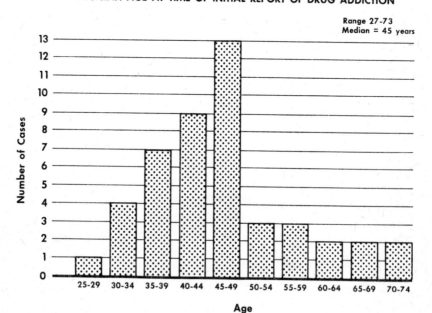

Range 27-73
Median = 45 years

Age

TABLE 3-V

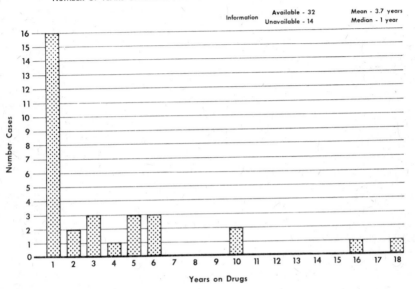

NUMBER OF YEARS ON DRUGS PRIOR TO STATE BOARD OF MEDICINE INITIAL ACTION

tive interview techniques on ninety-eight physician addicts, noted a negative attitude toward being a physician, a passive personality, and some feelings of omnipotence.

In a detailed study of thirty-six physician addicts, Wall[4] noted the following personality traits: sensitivity and tender-mindedness, with a tendency to hypochondriasis; easy fatigability and an inability to withstand stress; immaturity, inadequacy, and withdrawal; neurasthenia, depression, and "schizoid" make-up.

Modlin and Montes[5] felt that addiction in their physician patients was a symptom of moderately severe, progressive personality disorganization. Hill, Haertzen, and Yamahiro[6] employed the Minnesota Multiphasic Personality Inventory (MMPI) as a standard test on forty-two physician addicts and found strong evidence of general maladjustment, reflected as hypochondriasis, depression, general neuroticism, and anxiety.

TABLE 3-VI

PSYCHIATRIC DIAGNOSIS IN 31 CASES

Neuroses		Personality Disorders		Psychoses	
Depression	11	Passive Aggressive	5	Schizophrenia	4
Anxiety State	1	Compulsive	2	Paranoia	1
Transient Disorder	1	Others	2	Manic Depressive	2
				Chronic Brain Syndrome	2
	—		—		—
Totals	13		9		9

TABLE 3-VII

TYPICAL PROFILE OF DRUG-ADDICTED
PHYSICIANS REPORTED TO
VIRGINIA STATE BOARD OF MEDICINE

Graduate of a Virginia medical school
Speciality: General practice or internal medicine
White male
In practice: 18 years
Age at onset: 43 years
On drugs: 1-2 years
Principal drug used: Demerol®
Age at discovery: 45
Factors contributing to addiction
  (a) Chronic illness with pain
  (b) Family tragedy
  (c) Situational stress
  (d) Overwork
Discovered and reported by State Board of
  Pharmacy inspector
Psychiatric diagnosis: Depression

It has been generally accepted that some precipitating factor superimposed on a personality disorganization is an important key to the typical pattern of addiction. Our cases have shown that chronic illness and pain seem to be the most frequent precipitating causes of self-administration of drugs by physicians. The second most common precipitating factor is a tragic event, usually a family death. The third most commonly noted finding is that of a wife who becomes addicted, usually as a result of chronic painful illness (Table 3-VIII). It is frequently noted that the physician husband has been the provider of narcotics for his wife and has taken over the primary care of his spouse's illness. The psychiatric interplay in this combination of husband-and-wife drug addiction is truly complex. Needless to say, the finding of drug dependency in a physician's wife should be a cause for concern, with or without suspicious circumstances relating to the husband. Additional factors such as situational stress were also noted and, finally, overwork. The latter is often quoted in the literature as the most frequent causative factor, but in our experience it has not been a pre-

TABLE 3-VIII

ASSUMED PRECIPITATING FACTORS
FROM HISTORIES OF ADDICTED PHYSICIANS

Illness with physical pain	8
Tragedy	6
Addicted wife	5
Situational stress	5
Overwork	4
Marital problems	1
Information available (cases)	22

dominant finding.

The easy availability of drugs is, of course, a factor in physician drug addiction. Also, an attitude exists among physicians that because they are knowledgable about drug action, they are less likely to become addicted. Most physicians share the illusion that if they do begin to use drugs they can stop at once.

In most instances, the selection of a particular addicting drug is predictable. Our experience and that of others indicates that in recent years meperidine (Demerol®) has become the most frequently used addicting agent, with morphine the next most often abused. In earlier studies, morphine led as the drug of choice among addicted physicians. However, since Demerol was introducted in 1944, there has been a steady increase in its use by physicians as an addicting agent. This is partly due to the fact that Demerol was initially introduced as a nonaddictive drug, despite early warnings by Van Brucke[7] and Kucker.[8] In 1953, Isbell and White[9] called attention to the high incidence of Demerol addiction in nurses and physicians. Nevertheless, the idea still exists that because Demerol is a synthetic product, it is not a serious habit-forming drug. In fact, Demerol has been shown to be a major addictive agent in that it acts more rapidly

TABLE 3-IX

DRUGS MOST COMMONLY USED — ALONE OR IN COMBINATION

Demerol®	31	Pantopon®	2
Morphine	9	Tranquilizers	2
Dilaudid®	8	Opium	1
Amphetamine	7	Cocaine	1
Barbiturates	6	Paraldehyde	1
Talwin®	3	Leritine™	1
Methadone	3	Alcohol *never primary*	10
Codeine	2		

to produce greater elation with a shorter duration of effect than other drugs, particularly morphine. These characteristics of Demerol and its availability provide ideal conditions for addiction. Other drugs used by physician addicts in our study are listed in Table 3-IX. In some cases, alcohol was used in combination with drugs. This was also observed by Duffy and Litin,[10] who noted that many physicians went from alcoholism to drug addiction; once their drug addiction became established, the use of alcohol was discontinued.

Recently we and others have noted that pentazocine (Talwin®), a schedule VI drug, has become a frequent addicting agent among physicians.[11] Unfortunately, this drug is available without a federal narcotics permit, making control or its use more difficult.

Although it is difficult to categorize all drug-addicted physicians according to a single behavior pattern, their general activities have many similarities. The following cases are typical of addicted physicians:

Case 1: Doctor A. was a forty-six-year old, male general practitioner, married, with two children, living in a small rural community. He graduated from his state university medical school in the upper 10 percent of his class. He was extremely conscientious, carried a heavy workload, and seldom took a vacation, claiming his patients could not get along without him. He spent very little time with his family and left most of his child-rearing responsibilities to his wife. He felt that his childhood was marred by a weak, indecisive father and a demanding aggressive mother.

Doctor A. had little professional or social contact with any colleagues in his community. For many years he had suffered recurrent abdominal pain which was diagnosed as due to a severe irritable bowel syndrome. The pain became intense under excessive stress and prolonged periods of work. During one period of an exceptionally heavy workload, this physician could find little relief from this abdominal pain and, in order to continue working, gave himself an injection of 50 mg Demerol. He noted prompt and remarkable relief from the abdominal pain and a sense of well-being beyond any he had previously experienced. This initial self-injection of Demerol was soon followed by others. During the following six months, progressive changes were noted in Doctor A. He was no longer meticulous in his work; his medical decisions and judgment becamed flawed; his attitude toward patients changed from overconcern to disinterest. He reduced his previous prodigious workload to the point that he no longer saw many of his patients, and when he did see them, he talked at length of irrelevant matters. He became even more of a recluse, changing his schedule to night office hours and spending much of the day in futile paperwork of little consequence. He aroused the suspicions of his local pharmacist when he began ordering large quantities of Demerol for office use, far in excess of his previous supply. In addition, he often brought in prescriptions for Demerol for patients and said he would deliver the drug himself. During this period it became common knowledge, first among his colleagues and later in his community, that something was drastically wrong. A routine inspection by a state pharmacy inspector resulted in the exposure of Doctor A. as being addicted to Demerol.

Case 2: Doctor B. was a forty-four-year old, successful general surgeon who received his specialty training at a fine medical center in the East. He was chief of surgery of the 300-bed hospital where he worked. He was married to a woman whose family was socially prominent, and he was professionally and financially successful. He was perfectionistic in his work and demanding of himself and of those who worked with him. His workload was heavy, and he took pride in always being available at any time, day or night, that his patients needed him. Since childhood Doctor B. had suffered from severe migraine headaches and periods of depression. He frequently found that these attacks compromised his best surgical efforts and noted that the migraine often followed periods of increased tension. He also found that alcohol seemed to alleviate the headaches. Over a two-year period, Doctor B's colleagues noted that he frequently had alcohol on his breath while making hospital rounds. On several occasions, the night surgical supervisor reported that during phone calls, Doctor B's speech was slurred and his thinking seemed inconsistent. At social events it was often obvious that he had overindulged in alcohol. Despite his use of alcohol, the frequency of his migraine headaches increased. During a particularly severe attack one night, he was called to the hospital emergency room to perform an appendectomy on the son of a good friend. In order to function, he gave himself an injection of Demerol from the supply in his medical bag. There was a dramatic improvement in his headache, and he was able to perform the appendectomy without difficulty. After this episode, Demerol became a constant remedy for his migraine, and soon the slightest tension or frustration was an excuse for self-administration of the drug.

Before long, Doctor B.'s hospital behavior became a source of concern to his colleagues. His once consistent surgical performance became erratic; his surgical complications increased, and several unexplained deaths occurred among his patients. His former pattern of patient rounds changed, and frequently he was seen in the early morning hours making routine postsurgical visits. His previous busy social schedule also changed, and he gradually stopped seeing his many friends. His hospital chart entries became rambly and excessively long. It was reported on several occasions that he insisted on giving his patients their Demerol injections himself, and a number of times quantities of the drug were missing from the emergency room after one of his visits. Finally, after two unjustifiable postoperative deaths and continuing reports of a Demerol shortage in the hospital, Doctor B. was confronted by his colleagues about his addiction problem, which subsequent investigation confirmed.

Once his peers have recognized that a physician is addicted to drugs, what steps should be taken? First and foremost, the physician addict's hospital privileges should be suspended promptly, and a report made to the state board of medicine. Attempts at managing such a problem at the local level almost always fail.

Local disciplinary bodies seldom understand the devious behavior of addicted physicians and do not realize that drug addiction is a manifestation of severe mental illness. When apprehended, most addicted physicians will insist that they are able to stop their habit and only want an opportunity to try.

This triumph of hope over experience is doomed to failure. Those physicians urged to seek therapy on their own seldom do more than give lip service to such suggestions. Although they may appear to show both physical and mental improvement, almost invariably they regress or resort to a common alternative to addiction — that is, suicide.

It must be realized that treatment of the drug-addicted physician is a matter of years. Even when such a physician has psychiatric treatment in his local community, it is unusual for voluntary treatment to be effective for long, and even more unusual for the treating psychiatrist to report other than an optimistic prognosis to a hospital disciplinary committee. The result is the return of an incompletely treated physician to his previous life pattern, with almost universal failure in the cure of his addiction.

Why do we in Virginia urge that every addicted physician be reported to the state board of medicine? We do this because, over the years, we have developed a rehabilitation program that has restored 72 percent of physician addicts to medical practice (Table 3-X). Under this program, the addicted physician must immediately surrender his narcotics license — usually for life. His license to practice is placed on probationary status, and he must discontinue his practice. He is also required to appear for evaluation by the board's Psychiatric Advisory Committee. This committee, which is appointed by the Virginia State

TABLE 3-X

FINAL STATUS OF 46 DRUG-ADDICTED PHYSICIANS
REPORTED TO VIRGINIA STATE BOARD OF MEDICINE

Number Returning to Practice	33
Private	27
Institutional	6
Number Not Returning to Practice	13
License Revoked	11
Left State	2
Rehabilitated	72%

Board of Medicine is responsible for interviewing and evaluating the mental status of physicians referred to it by the Board.

The physician must then seek psychiatric and medical care. This care may be of his own choosing, but it must be approved by the Psychiatric Advisory Committee. The physician's progress and condition are monitored by the committee through regular interviews, by reports from the treating psychiatrist, and by mandatory periodic return visits before the entire board.

When the addicted physician's treating psychiatrist, the board's Psychiatric Advisory Committee, and the State Board of Medicine feel he is ready to return to practice, permission is granted for a limited work schedule, often in a protected environment. With constant surveillance and repeated interviews by the board and the Psychiatric Advisory Committee, the addicted physician is gradually guided back into full practice responsibility. Unfortunately, not all physician addicts respond to this regimen and relapses are frequent; some never recover.

In addition to the forty-six physician addicts in our study, the Virginia board has handled an additional eighteen physician addicts who were reported in the second and third quarters of 1974,[3] in 1975, [6] and in 1976.[9] The profile of these additional eighteen cases is remarkably similar to that described in our study.

REFERENCES

1. Anslinger, H. J.: Interview. *Mod Med Annual, 25*:975-982, 1957.
2. Green, R. C., Carroll, G., and Buxton, D.: Drug addiction among physicians; the Virginia experience. *JAMA, 236*:12, 1372-1375, 1976.
3. Winick, C.: Physician narcotic addicts. *Soc Probl, 9*:174-186, 1961.
4. Wall, J. H.: The results of hospital treatment of addiction in physicians. *Federation Bull, 45*:144-152, 1958.
5. Modlin, H. C., and Montes, A.: Narcotic addiction in physicians. *Am J Psychiatry, 121*:358-365, 1964.
6. Hill, H. E., Haertzen, C. A., and Yamahiro, R. S.: The addict physician: a Minnesota Multiphasic Personality Inventory study of the interaction of personality characteristics and availability of narcotics. *Res Publ Assoc Res Nerv Ment Dis, 46*:321-332, 1966.

7. von Brucke, S.: Ueber Dolantinabusus und einen Fall von Dolantindelir. *Wein Klin Wochenschr, 52*:854, 1940.

8. Kucker, I.: Zwei Falle von Dolantinsucht. *Wein Klin Wochenschr, 19*:688, 1942.

9. Isbell, H. and White, W. M.: Symposium on drug addiction: clinical characteristics of addictions. *Am J Med, 14*:558-565, 1953.

10. Duffy, J. C. and Litin, E. M.: *The Emotional Health of Physicians.* Springfield, Ill., Charles C Thomas Publisher, 63, 1967.

11. Editorial: Pentazocine a "non-addicting" drug. *Federation Bull, 57*:78, 1970.

Chapter 4

ALCOHOLISM AMONG PHYSICIANS

IT is a truism that alcoholism occurs among all types of people in our society, including doctors of medicine. Although this is not a new situation, we believe it is now one factor among many that may account for the lowered public esteem of the medical profession. More importantly, alcoholism among physicians results at times in poor or inadequate care of patients.

Abuse of alcohol is difficult to define with precision. It has been said that "there are almost as many definitions of alcoholism as there are alcoholics." For our purposes, we are using the definition set forth in the American Medical Association's *Manual on Alcoholism:*[1]

> Alcoholism is an illness characterized by preoccupation with alcohol and loss of control over its consumption, such as to usually lead to intoxication if drinking is begun; by chronicity; by progression; and by a tendency toward relapse. It is particularly associated with physical disability and impaired emotional, occupational, and/or social adjustments as a direct consequence of persistent and excessive use of alcohol.

This rather broad definition is useful because it not only covers the adverse consequences of excessive drinking but also includes the key factor of "loss of control." Complete loss of control of alcohol consumption indicates that the alcoholic must forever strive to maintain total abstinence. If a measure of control remains, the excessive drinker may still be able to moderate his drinking habit without necessarily remaining fully abstinent. Although a distinction is thus made between alcoholism and excessive drinking, it should be borne in mind that both situations may be equally deleterious to the proper practice of medicine. One must also remember that alcoholism is usually preceded by many years of progressively increasing excessive use of alcohol.

Additional objective signs of the prodromal phase of alcohol addiction according to Jellinek[2] include amnesia or "black-outs" occurring as a result of only "moderate" alcohol intake; surreptitious drinking, often associated with hastily imbibing a few drinks and subsequent early onset of intoxication; a preoccupation with alcohol such as concern over having an "adequate" supply available; a fear of "running out" or "not having enough" for the next day; and an avoidance of verbal references to alcohol such as jokes about it in relation to the individual affected or others. Jellinek also pointed out that onset of the critical phase of alcoholism is signalled by the start of "loss of control." All physicians should be familiar with these and other symptoms discussed by Jellinek in order to facilitate recognition of potential or actual alcoholism in their patients, their colleagues, and, possibly, in themselves.

As the problem of alcoholism in a physician progresses, various changes in personality and work habits may be observed. There may be social isolation or withdrawal from friends and associates. A formerly conscientious physician may become unavailable, especially on weekends, so that his patients must call another doctor. Although less obvious than among industrial workers, "Monday morning absences" become part of the alcoholic physician's behavioral pattern. He also starts to call his office saying he is "sick" or goes to work "not feeling very well" and leaves early, canceling appointments. The formerly busy and overworked doctor is "away" with increasing frequency, and he spends more and more time "on vacation" or literally hides at a country place. Office personnel as well as family often assist in these coverups or excuses out of loyalty, fear of exposure, or fear of retaliation.

Colleagues and patients may note irregularly kept hours, decreasing efficiency, forgetfulness, broken promises, and a deterioration in handwriting. Increasingly, colleagues are asked to cover the alcoholic physician's calls for various reasons except the real one. Patients may note inattention, lack of thoroughness, impatience to end a visit, or failure to give proper treatment. Consultations or referrals decrease markedly or become inappropriate. Consultants may find inadequate records or, sometimes, diffuse reports that are not particularly pertinent to the immediate problem as well as a lack of seemingly obvious proper treatment. Patients may be discharged prematurely or kept in the hospital longer than necessary.

Peer review or hospital utilization committees should recognize and act in such cases, but often they do little or nothing unless the circumstances are too blatant to ignore. Eventually the alcoholic physician may try to work while still "under the influence," even when intoxication or an odor of alcohol is evident to everyone except apparently the doctor himself. In due course, patients will change doctors, fewer new patients will appear, and the entire practice and income will decrease sharply. Finally, the hospital staff may be forced to take action by suspending hospital privileges, but medical societies rarely intervene. Many times, however, a hospital stay only means "drying out" or treatment of acute symptoms without establishing chronic alcoholism as the basic problem.

The alcoholic physician rarely seeks help before his problem becomes critical. When alcoholic doctors do look for assistance, they usually consult psychiatrists.[3] Most general physicians do not like to cope with alcoholism, and this is also true of some psychiatrists. The reasons for this, we believe, include a lack of sufficient attention to alcoholism in medical school curricula, a mistaken idea that prognosis in alcoholism is always poor, and an inability to anticipate and tolerate alcoholic patients' relapses during treatment. (Few alcoholics achieve permanent abstinence right from the start of treatment.)

What should be done when a physician becomes an alcoholic or has an obvious drinking problem? If the situation is recognized by the alcoholic doctor's own physician, the latter should confront the patient directly. The attending physician should be kind but factual and frank as to the immediate or anticipated consequences. He should also offer helpful information on facilities available for treatment and counsel and should inform his physician-patient about the program of Alcoholics Anonymous. In some cases it may be valuable to have the patient's wife present during such a discussion. If the attending physician is hesitant to act alone, we suggest that he ask two or three of his colleagues to join him when he first confronts the affected physician. The presence of several professional friends may help to counter the alcoholic's tendency to deny, belittle, or excuse his problem. A favorable outcome of treatment should be stressed because, despite denials, the alcoholic physician may be depressed, seriously concerned for his future, and secretly feel a sense of hopelessness.

In some cases alcoholic physicians who do not seek treatment on their own initiative must undergo involuntary commitment to a state or private hospital. Unless a hospital has a special program for alcoholics which, ideally, should include involvement with Alcoholics Anonymous, hospitalization may be of little benefit. Adequate posthospital treatment on a continuing basis is absolutely necessary to maintain sobriety.

Loss of hospital privileges or censure by a medical society may indicate the seriousness of the alcoholic physician's problem, but they do not prevent his continuing to practice medicine. The privilege to practice ultimately rests with the state licensing board. Such boards should be notified whenever a physician is suspected of abusing alcohol. The board should investigate, evaluate the situation, and then take whatever steps are appropriate for the public's protection. Next should come a program of rehabilitation as outlined in Chapter 3.

When considering the statistics cited below, several factors must be borne in mind. Many reports do not cite comparable figures, i.e. incidence of alcoholism may be based on surveys or simply the authors' estimates. Some report incidence of physicians among hospitalized alcoholics, others the number of alcoholic physicians among physicians hospitalized for psychiatric treatment.

Accurate figures on the incidence of alcoholism are not available, but it is estimated that nationally there are from 4.5 to 6 million adult Americans who may be classified as alcoholics.[4, 5] Cahalan and Cisin[6] estimated that 9 percent of a national probability sample of drinkers they studied represented persons who by definition would be considered alcoholics. If this percentage is projected to the 1974 figure of 379,748 physicians in the continental United States, Alaska, Hawaii, and protectorate territories,[7] there were 23,924 (in 1974) physicians in all categories who would have met the criteria for classification as alcoholics.

As social attitudes have become less judgmental in recent years, such euphemisms as "the problem drinker" or "misuser of alcohol" have become common rather than the more absolute definition of alcoholism formulated by the AMA. Straus[8] pointed out that, since 1940, the "perceived" percentage of alcohol users has increased by 15 percent, and the number of "problem" users has risen to a total of 4 or 5 percent of the total population. Lipp and Benson[9] found only 8 percent of a physician sample to be total abstainers as compared with 32 percent of all adults estimated as abstainers in a survey by Cahalan and Cisin.[6] Studies by Glatt[10] of male alcoholics in two British hospitals showed an incidence of 3.8 and 3.0 percent doctors. Glatt also reported a higher incidence of cirrhosis of the liver in British doctors as compared with the general population. In the British studies, alcoholism was found to occur more often than drug addiction among British physicians.

Other studies[11-13] showed alcoholism to be the second most frequent diagnosis in physicians hospitalized for all psychiatric reasons, the first being drug addiction. A 1973 report of the AMA Council on Mental Health[14] stated that the Arizona State Board of Medical Examiners disciplined 3.2 percent of physicians over an eleven-year period for alcoholism. That same report showed that in Oregon, the rate was 2.3 percent for alcoholism over a ten-year period.

Reports[13-15] have also pointed out that alcoholism among physicians not only may precede drug addiction but often is associated with the use of one or more mood-altering or analgesic drugs. When used with alcohol, drugs obviously intensify an already serious problem.

Over a ten-year period, 1967 to 1976, the Virginia State Board of Medicine handled fifteen cases of alcoholic physicians. As the average number of physicians licensed in Virginia during this period was 5,660, the alcoholic physicians reported to the board represented only 0.27 percent of all licensed physicians in the state. No more than three cases were reported in any year, and in most years, there were only two cases or none reported. It should also be noted that as the total number of licensed physicians increased, there was no corresponding increase in reported cases of alcoholism. Such statistics arouse concern about alcoholic doctors who remain officially undetected.

All the alcoholic physicians reported in Virginia were male. Their average age when brought to the attention of the board was fifty-four years. Their average age at graduation from medical school was twenty-seven years. (The duration of true alcoholism is unknown in most cases.)

Board actions most often consisted of placing the doctor's license on probation, with the stipulation that he work only in a supervised situation, such as in a state mental hospital. Additional probationary requirements were that the alcoholic physician undergo treatment, attend Alcoholics Anonymous, or continue with Antabuse®, if prescribed by his therapist. The therapists were obliged to report to the board at intervals. Failure to meet the conditions of probation led to the revocation of license. In some cases, such requirements of the board may have a beneficial effect on the outcome.

In this series of alcoholic physicians, one-third also gave a history of drug dependence, most often with minor tranquilizers and analgesics. It should be emphasized, however, that drug addiction per se was not the primary problem at the time these physicians were seen by the board, even though in a few cases the reported physician's narcotic license had been revoked because of misuse of narcotics.

Definitive results of studies of alcoholics are difficult to obtain because there may be sobriety for a period of years, only to be followed by relapse. Good results are defined as sobriety and a demonstrated ability to function well for one or more years. Poor results include continued use of alcohol and inability to function well. According to these criteria, of the fifteen cases available to follow-up, six or 40 percent showed good results; four or 27 percent showed poor results; in five or 33 percent of cases, results are unknown. Four of the physicians in this group had died and three had retired at the time of this review. Evaluation of these seven cases was made when those events occurred. Only four doctors in the study currently hold Virginia licenses.

Five of the physicians reported were known to have affiliated with Alcoholics Anonymous, and four of these showed good results.

REFERENCES

1. American Medical Association: *Manual on Alcoholism.* Chicago, 3, 1973.
2. Jellinek, E. M.: Phases of alcohol addiction. *Q J Stud Alcohol, 13*:678-679, 1952.
3. Bissell, L. C. and Jones, R. W.: The alcoholic physician: a survey. *Am J Psychiatry, 133*:1142-1145, 1976.
4. *Alcohol and Alcoholism. Publication #1640,* U.S. Department of Health, Education, and Welfare, 10, 1967.
5. Keller, M.: The definition of alcoholism and the estimation of its prevalence. In Pittman, D. J. and Snyder, C. R., (Ed.): *Society, Culture and Drinking Patterns.* New York, John Wiley & Sons, 1962.
6. Cahalan, D. and Cisin, I. H.: American drinking practices: summary of findings from a national probability sample. *Q J Stud Alcohol, 29*:130-151, 1968.
7. *Profile of Medical Practice 1975.* Chicago, AMA Center for Health Services and Development, 75, 1976.
8. Straus, R.: Problem drinking in the perspective of social change. In Filstead, W. J., Rossi, J. J., and Keller, M., (Ed.): *Alcohol and Alcohol Problems: New Thinking and New Directions.* Cambridge, Ballinger Publishing Company, 41, 1976.
9. Lipp, M. R. and Benson, S. G.: Physician use of marijuana, alcohol, and tobacco. *Am J Psychiatry, 129*:612-616, 1972.
10. Glatt, M. M.: Alcoholism among doctors. *Lancet, 2*:342-343, 1974.
11. Duffy, J. C. and Litin, E. M.: Psychiatric morbidity of physicians. *JAMA, 189*:989-992, 1964.
12. Pearson, M. M. and Streaker, E. A.: Physicians as psychiatric patients: private practice experience. *Am J Psychiatry, 116*:915-919, 1960.
13. Vincent, M. O., Robinson, E. A., and Latt, L.: Physicians as patients: private psychiatric hospital experiences. *Can Med Assoc J, 100*:403-412, 1969.
14. AMA Council on Mental Health: The sick physician; impairment by psychiatric disorders, including alcoholism and drug dependence. *JAMA, 223*:684-687, 1973.

15. Bissell, L. C. and Mooney, A. J.: The special problem of the alcoholic physician. *Med Times, 103*:63-73, 1975.

Chapter 5

PSYCHIATRIC ILLNESS
AMONG PHYSICIANS

PHYSICIANS are no more immune from psychiatric disorders than from physical illness. Indeed, there is some thought that psychiatric problems among members of the medical profession are more prevalent than in other professions or even in the general population. In discussing this aspect of physician impairment, we exclude the chemical addiction and senility which are dealt with elsewhere in this book.

In this chapter, we will focus attention on factors which may be involved in the frequency of suicide and psychiatric illness as well as the most prevalent psychiatric diagnosis among physicians. We will also discuss our own experience with psychiatrically impaired physicians.

Waring[1] concluded that accurate statistics on psychiatric disorders in doctors of medicine are unobtainable. This is so because of varying methods of reporting, lack of controls, and uncertainty about the actual incidence of such disorders in the general population. As noted, some reports include psychiatric illnesses with drug abuse. Others refer to "visits to the psychiatrist," while still others list psychiatric diagnoses based on hospitalization. When questionnaires are used, it is difficult to know how to classify nonrespondents.

Disciplinary actions by state boards of medical examiners obviously do not reflect a true incidence of mental illness among doctors, but they do suggest the significance of the problem. In 1973, the AMA Council on Mental Health[2] reported figures from the state boards in Arizona and Oregon. For periods of eleven and ten years, respectively, these two states reported disciplinary actions against 1.3 (Arizona) and 0.9 (Oregon) percent of practicing physicians. These actions were taken because of mental disorders other than alcoholism or drug dependency, both of which occurred more often.

Pearson and Streaker,[3] in 1969, pointed out that physicians were much more likely to seek private rather than public psychiatric care if they became ill. As evidence, they noted that among admissions to two Philadelphia hospitals in 1958, only 0.05 percent represented physicians admitted to the public institution, while 2.7 percent of admissions to a private hospital were doctors. They also reported that of all private patients seen by one author over a fifteen-year period, only 3 percent were physicians.

In a 1964 survey of a seven-year period, 1956 to 1963, Duffy and Litin[4] reported that of 5,925 admissions to the psychiatric service of the Mayo Clinic, 93 were physicians. This represents a ratio of one doctor in every sixty-four admissions, or 1.6 percent. Here the ratio of physician-patients is much higher than the proportion of physicians in the general population. The authors did not indicate the location of practice of the physician-patients, but they did write, "Many physicians come to our institution because the safe distance from home assures a measure of anonymity, and because ours is not identified as primarily a psychiatric center." The fact that the Mayo Clinic and the two hospitals to which its staff admit patients are private institutions may also help to explain a higher concentration of physician-patients.

In a 1967 report, a'Brook, Hailstone, and McLauchlan[5] discussed 192 doctors seen because of psychiatric illness in the ten years from 1954 to 1964. This study involved two British Hospitals and included both inpatients and outpatients, 114 and 78, respectively. At one hospital doctors represented one of every eighty-two admissions, or 1.2 percent; at the second hospital, the rate was one doctor for every forty-three admissions, or 2.3 percent. When chemical dependency is omitted, the figures showed that 0.79 percent of patients admitted to the two hospitals during the study period were physicians.

Small et al.[6], in a 1969 publication, reported on forty physician psychiatric inpatients over a thirteen-year period from 1952 to 1965. These doctors accounted for one of every 130 psychiatric hospital admissions, or 0.77 percent. Only twenty-seven of these forty physicians were diagnosed as mentally ill, the rest of the diagnoses were alcohol or drug related. These twenty-seven would make a ratio of 1 to 193 admissions, or 0.52 percent being mentally ill.

According to Vincent, Robinson, and Latt[7], in a 1969 report on a seven-year period, 1960 to 1967, ninety-three physicians were among patients admitted to a private psychiatric hospital. The authors state that this equalled a ratio of one physician for every forty-four first admissions for psychiatric problems, or 2.3 percent. As fifty-three of these ninety-three physicians had drug or alcohol problems, then only forty would be considered mentally ill as used in this chapter. These forty mentally ill physicians would constitute a ratio of 1 to 102 admissions or 0.98 percent.

A more recent study by Vaillant, Sobowale, and McArthur[8], in 1972, was concerned primarily with the psychologic histories of a selected group of physicians. Of forty-six physicians followed for thirty years after their sophomore year in college, 34 percent reported ten or more visits to a psychiatrist. This was a significantly higher figure than for a control group of comparable socioeconomic status. Hospitalization for psychiatric causes occurred in 17 percent of the physicians, but in only 6 percent of the controls; this comparison, however, was not considered statistically significant.

The number of studies to date is small for both inpatient and outpatient physicians in whom psychiatric disorders have been reported, but the numerical similarities among the studies are remarkable. Also, the hospitalization figures available from the United States, Canada, and England show little variation. It should be emphasized that these statistics reflect only the experience of private institutions. Information about admissions to state or public hospitals, with the exception of the Pearson and Strecker[3] report, is unavailable.

In the studies discussed here, cases of alcoholism and drug dependency are usually included with other psychiatric diagnoses. On this basis, the figures are again similar and show an average of 1.53 percent of all psychiatric admissions to be physicians. This suggests that when chemical addiction is included with other conditions, it accounts for about one half of the total psychiatric cases among physicians.

From 1967 to 1976, the Virginia State Board of Medicine identified twenty-one physicians with "psychiatric disorders," as defined in this chapter. During this ten-year period, the number of doctors licensed to practice in the state averaged 5,600. The twenty-one physicians thus represented only 0.38 percent of their colleagues.

Of the twenty-one Virginia physicians with psychiatric disorders, all were males except one. Their ages ranged from 36 to 60 years, with an average age of 46.5 years when brought to the board's attention. The largest single group were general practitioners (28%), with psychiatrists next (19%).

The relatively high percentage of psychiatrists is related in part to certain questions on the state's licensing application forms. Applicants are asked not only about any history of mental illness, alcoholism, and drug problems, but also if they have ever received psychotherapy. Board inquiries about affirmative answers regarding therapy revealed that a major proportion of the respondents were psychiatrists who had had psychotherapy as part of their specialty training. In most cases, the follow-up was resolved by correspondence. In the 7 percent of such instances in which some doubts remained, the applicants were interviewed in person by the board's Psychiatric Advisory Committee. In four cases, it was felt that "a personality problem" existed, but all were granted licenses to practice. In the majority of cases, the committee did not establish any definable psychiatric diagnosis. The licensure question about psychotherapy proved to be unproductive and is no longer included on the application form.

Three of the twenty-one physicians in the study were admitted to a state hospital because of "mental illness," but no further information was available on them. Diagnoses in the remaining eighteen cases were as follows: personality disorders, ten (56%); psychoses, six (33%); and neuroses, two (11%).

In only three (16%) cases did the physicians involved give a history of difficulty with alcohol or drugs.

Follow-up information is inadequate for approximately 50 percent of cases. Of the remaining, eleven physicians had valid

Virginia licenses in 1976 and have been reported as functioning well. In nine cases the physicians did not have a Virginia license, and death occurred in one case.

It should be obvious that state board statistics do not reflect a true incidence of psychiatric illnesses. The boards usually are not made aware of a physician's psychiatric problems until major malfunction has occurred or a doctor has been involuntarily committed to a state hospital. Percentages of physicians reported by state boards vary from state to state. Arizona[2] reported 1.3 percent disciplinary actions for psychiatric causes while the Virginia figure was 0.38 percent. Derbyshire[9], reporting on all types of disciplinary actions by examining boards throughout the United States, cites variation ranging from 0.11 to 2.0 percent.

At the second AMA conference on "The Impaired Physician," in Atlanta in February 1977, it was clear that most state boards never learn of the psychiatric or other disabling problems affecting physicians. Currently, in many states, means are available through state medical societies to reach and assist sick doctors without involving the state medical boards. In most cases treatment is confidential and unrecorded.

Several states now have statutes requiring that physicians who are under psychiatric treatment be reported to the state board. These are relatively new laws, and their effectiveness is still unknown. The reporting requirements may well identify a greater number of physicians with psychiatric disorders, but they may lead doctors to avoid treatment or to seek it "out-of-state" to avoid detection.

Figures cited on the incidence of physicians among psychiatric inpatients suggest a higher ratio than in the general population. However, we do not know to what extent doctors may have been concentrated in the few hospitals for which statistics are available. Until many more studies are made, taking into account residence, physician-to-population ratios, total physicians, etc., we will not have adequate data. Information is also needed on psychiatric problems handled on an outpatient, as well as inpatient basis. More physicians are probably treated as outpatients than on an inpatient basis but, again, valid statistics are unavailable. Outpatient care can, of course, be very successful, even for severe psychiatric disorders.

Over a fifteen-year period, Pearson[3] saw seventy-one physician patients who constituted about 3 percent of his private patients. Of sixty-six of these physicians on whom reports were made, two-thirds were outpatients. There is no way to know if the experience of this author is typical or if he treated more physicians than other psychiatrists.

a'Brook and associates[5] reported 78 physician outpatients and 114 inpatients, but no projections are possible from these figures. Results of treatment were very similar in the two groups, as were the conditions affecting them. An exception was that there were more suicides among the inpatients. It was noted, too, that more surgeons were inpatients and more psychiatrists were outpatients. Of the forty-six cases reported by Vaillant and associates,[8] 34 percent received outpatient treatment.

Although data from these studies are somewhat meager and vary considerably, they tend to confirm that psychiatric illness may occur more often in physicians than in the general population or in other professional groups. However, this is again merely an assumption, as the data are not sufficiently comprehensive for accurate comparisons.

Psychiatric diagnostic categories in the five reports cited,[3-7] which cover a total of 484 physicians, are as follows:

Diagnosis	Total Average (Percent)
Affective Psychoses	20
Personality Disorders	8
Neuroses	14
Schizophrenia	16*
Organic Disorders	3
Chemical Addictions	39†

*Figure is somewhat elevated by one report[6] in which this diagnosis represented 53 percent of cases. The average of the other four reports was only 6 percent schizophrenia.
†Figure represents some personality disorders with addiction in some reports, but not in others.

In general, the most frequent psychiatric illnesses reported are the affective disorders, mainly depressive in nature. Some studies list personality disorders in place of addiction, thus raising the percentage figure for this diagnosis.

The three most common psychiatric problems found in the studies cited were (1) drug addiction, (2) alcoholism, and (3) depression, respectively.

What factors account for the psychiatric morbidity of physicians? Many physician patients blame their illness on overwork; however, all overworked doctors do not become ill. Also physicians are not alone in being overworked. Although Cramond[10] found that clinicians are more prone to anxiety states than nonclinicians, other studies[5, 6] have shown that industrial, public health, institutional, and academic physicians are not entirely immune.

Vaillant et al.[8], in their prospective study, rated their subjects on childhood adjustment scores, showing that poor adjustment correlated with later psychiatric difficulties. Marital problems, as well as divorce, occur more often among impaired physicians. This, in turn, seems to lead to difficult adjustments for their children. As a considerable proportion of physicians are the children of physicians, the process may be perpetuated. One may also speculate on the role of hereditary factors. Various studies[11-13] of medical students and resident physicians have shown significant psychopathology in these subjects, lending support to Waring,[1] who stated that ". . . there seems to be overwhelming evidence that those physicians who develop psychiatric illness have a vulnerability that antedates medical school."

In this country suicide is commonly considered a manifestation of mental illness, most often some form of depression.[14] Suicide rates are also relatively high among alcoholics and drug addicts.[15-17] As the incidence of these disorders is comparatively high among physicians, a correspondingly high rate of suicide would be expected for this group and has been documented.[14, 18, 19] De Sole, Aronson, and Singer[14] estimated the suicide rate among physicians, from 1902 to 1910, to be 3.36 times the rate for the general population. Using *JAMA* obituaries from 1965 to 1968, they found 26 percent of all deaths occurring in physicians between the ages of twenty-five and thirty-nine years were the result of suicide. For all white males of the same age, 9 percent of all deaths were due to suicide. A 1968 study[17] of *JAMA* reports on 228 physician suicides showed that the rate of suicides among female physicians was double that among male physicians. Blachly, Disher, and Roduner[16] studied 200 suicides among physicians and found that 26 percent of physician suicides were under psychiatric care at the time of death. Of the 200, 39 percent were heavy drinkers or alcoholic and 19 percent were heavy users of drugs or were addicted to them. In contrast to other writers, these authors concluded, "Physicians do not commit suicide more frequently than persons in other professions such as law, dentistry or the military." Dublin and Spiegelman[20] also reported only a slightly higher suicide rate among physicians, 39.0 vs 37.6 per 100,000 for white males. When physicians do take their own lives, their average age is forty-eight years, but 50 percent were between thirty-five and fifty-four years old.[19] von Brauchitsch[21] also questioned the reported high rate of suicide among physicians.

Results of treatment of mentally ill doctors are difficult to evaluate. Some reports do not address this aspect at all; others approach it by various means; i.e. questionnaires, status of license to practice, type of hospital discharge, etc. One report may be optimistic,[6] another may stress the problem of treating a fellow physician.[5]

Small et al.[6] reviewed the records at Indiana University Hospital of a group of forty physicians hospitalized for psychiatric problems. They found discharge against medical advice in 12.5 percent of cases compared with 1.3 percent for psychiatric patients generally; follow-up periods averaged 9.3 years, ranging from 2.5 to 13 years; suicide occurred in five physicians (12.5%); three died of other causes; seven had repeated hospital admissions; eight were no longer practicing. For unexplained reasons, the number of patients in this series diagnosed as schizophrenic was high, 21 or 53 percent. In spite of the poor prognosis for this illness, 57 percent of physicians affected were actively practicing at time of follow-up. The overall percentage still practicing was in the same range.

Pearson and Streaker[3] reported on sixty-six physicians treated on both an outpatient (70%) and inpatient (30%) basis. Nineteen of the group were seen for "consultation only," and no treatment results were noted. Of the other forty-seven patients, twenty-eight (60%) were described as "much improved," while nineteen (40%) were "slightly improved," "not changed," or "worse." Presumably, these results were noted at time of discharge as subsequent follow-up was not reported.

The study by a'Brook et al.[5] covered 114 inpatients seen from January 1954 to January 1964. Of these, 8.6 percent were schizophrenic. Six (5.3%) committed suicide. In 1964, eighty (70.2%) were still registered to practice; thirty-four (29.8%) were no longer registered. However, of the eighty registered, fourteen were known to have discontinued practicing because of their illnesses, leaving 58 percent presumed to be practicing.

Despite the variations in diagnoses, the three studies[3, 5, 6] cited earlier indicate average "good" results in 58.3 percent of the study groups, which included alcoholism and drug addiction together with mental illness. If this figure (58.3%) is accurate, we must conclude that psychiatrically affected physicians have a fairly good prognosis.

REFERENCES

1. Waring, E. M.: Psychiatric illness in physicians: a review. *Compr Psychiatry, 15*:519-530, 1974.
2. AMA Council on Mental Health: Impairment by psychiatric disorders, including alcoholism and drug dependence. *JAMA, 223*:684-687, 1973.
3. Pearson, M. M. and Streaker, E. A.: Physicians as psychiatric patients: private practice experience. *Am J Psychiatry, 116*:915-919, 1969.
4. Duffy, J. C. and Litin, E. M.: Psychiatric morbidity of physicians. *JAMA, 189*:989-992, 1964.
5. a'Brook, M. F., Hailstone, J. D. and McLauchlan, I. E. J.: Psychiatric illness in the medical profession. *Br J Psychiatry, 113*:1013-1023, 1967.
6. Small, I. F., Small, J. G., Assuc, D. M., and Moore, D. F.: The fate of the mentally ill physician. *Am J Psychiatry, 125*:1333-1342, 1969.
7. Vincent, M. O., Robinson, E. A., and Latt, L.: Physicians as patients: private psychiatric hospital experience. *Can Med Assoc J, 100*:403-412, 1969.
8. Vaillant, G. E., Sobowale, N. C., and McArther, C.: Some psychologic

vulnerabilities of physicians. *N Engl J Med, 287*:372-375, 1972.

9. Derbyshire, R. C.: Medical ethics and discipline. *JAMA, 228*:59-62, 1974.

10. Cramond, W. A.: Anxiety in medical practice — the doctor's anxiety. *Aust NZ J Psychiatry, 3*:324-329, 1969.

11. Pitts, F. N., Jr., Winokur, G., and Steward, M. A.: Psychiatric syndromes, anxiety, symptoms, and responses to stress in medical students. *Am J Psychiatry, 118*:333-340, 1961.

12. Hunter, R. C. A., Lohrenz, J. G., and Schwartzman, A. E.: Nosophobia and hypochondriasis in medical students. *J Nerv Ment Dis, 139*:147-152, 1964.

13. Strecker, E. A., Appel, K. E., Palmer, H. D., and Braceland, F. J.: Psychiatric studies in medication; II: Neurotic trends in senior medical students. *Am J Psychiatry, 93*:1197-1229, 1937.

14. De Sole, D. E., Aronson, S., and Singer, P.: Suicide and role strain among physicians. *Int J Soc Psychiatry, 15*:294-301, 1969.

15. Wall, J. H.: The results of hospital treatment of addiction in physicians. *Federation Bull, 45*:144-152, 1958.

16. Blachly, P. H., Disher, W., and Roduner, G.: Suicide by physicians. *Bull Suicidology*, 1-18, Dec., 1968.

17. Craig, A. G. and Pitts, F. N.: Suicide by physicians. *Dis Nerv Syst, 29*:763-772, 1968.

18. Ross, M.: Suicide among physicians. A psychological study. *Dis Nerv Syst, 34*:145-150, 1973.

19. Rose, K. D. and Rosow, I.: Physicians who kill themselves. *Arch Gen Psychiatry, 29*:800-805, 1973.

20. Dublin, L. I. and Spiegelman, M.: The longevity and mortality of American physicians, 1938-1942; preliminary report. *JAMA, 134*:1211-1215, 1947.

21. von Brauchitsch, H.: The physician suicide revisited. *J Nerv Ment Dis, 162*:40-45, 1976.

Chapter 6

BEHAVIORAL PROBLEMS
AMONG PHYSICIANS

IN the present context, behavioral problems among physicians may be categorized rather broadly to include indiscriminate use of drugs, senility, unprofessional conduct, incompetence, fraud, and abuse. With growing frequency, deviant behavior culminates in cases requiring disciplinary action on the part of state medical licensing boards. The number of cases of this type referred to the Virginia State Board of Medicine has been relatively small, except for indiscriminate use of drugs and alcohol. In general, low incidence of cases has been due primarily to the difficulty of identifying reportable behavioral problems. Within the last three or four years, however, the number of cases reported has increased, in part because of heightened sensitivity of hospital personnel and of the public and, in the state of Virginia, because of more effective investigative activity.

Since 1973, the Virginia State Board of Medicine has had the help of the Virginia Board of Pharmacy inspectors and, more recently, the medical board hired its own full-time inspector. Through this intensified effort, more cases of behavioral problems among doctors in the state have been brought to the medical board's attention.

When physical or mental disability prevents a doctor from caring for his patients adequately, compassion and sympathy for the affected doctor often supersede objective evaluation of his professional competence. When the consequences of aging, an injury, or a disease process have deleterious effects on a physician's ability to function well, primary consideration must be extended to his patients. A doctor who has a progressive tremor, indicating an underlying disorder, or one who too often forgets important details may commit serious errors in caring for patients, and it is essential that those patients be protected from such lapses.

It is extremely difficult, if not impossible, to determine accurately when a person becomes incapable of productive effort and when retirement should be encouraged or mandated. The Social Security Act of 1935 arbitrarily established age sixty-five as the year of eligibility for full benefits based on age. The Social Security system has been reasonably effective, but it has also forced many still healthy, productive, and potentially valuable people to retire prematurely. This has resulted in a loss not only to the persons concerned but also to the economy and to society generally. In addition, there is evidence, reported by the AMA Committee on Aging,[1] that forced retirement may accelerate the aging process. In medicine, this type of problem has been avoided to a degree in that there is no mandatory retirement age for a doctor in private practice. Although this latitude permits many talented and capable doctors to continue to practice well beyond a mandatory retirement age, it also makes it necessary for empowered medical bodies to determine competence and to restrain the doctor who can no longer perform adequately because of the effects of aging.

Duffy[2] has pointed out that in spite of continuous involvement with illness, injury, and disability, many physicians never consider the implications of physical disability in relation to themselves or their colleagues. Among the many complexities that must be considered is the affected doctor's emotional reaction to his situation. Although the extent and nature of his disability are important, often it is the emotional component that directly affects his practice.

When dealing with an impaired doctor, it is important to consider all available options. It is not always necessary to move immediately toward revocation of a license to practice. It may be feasible to arrange that the doctor in question continue to practice on a limited basis, under close supervision or with extensive assistance, thus utilizing his functional expertise and abilities. This course of action should always be considered and, if possible, implemented.

Senility is usually an insidious process, as are often the symptoms of many progressive disorders, and there may be no marked or dramatic signs of disability. Colleagues may become aware that a physician has begun to work more slowly or that he has become forgetful. Frequently, in fact, it is the hospital nursing staff that notices such signs first. For example, a surgeon may require more time than formerly to perform a familiar procedure. An operating room nurse notices this and reports it to her supervisor, who conveys the observation to the hospital's chief of surgery. If the problem persists, the hospital's medical staff ultimately must act, and the case is then referred to the institution's board of directors. It is at this point that such cases are usually presented to the state board of medicine. As noted, management of this type of case is difficult. The doctor's colleagues must strive to be sensitive, compassionate, and fair. Patients must be protected, but the physician should not be "forced to retire," if he still is able to practice safely in a restricted manner.

An example of a constructive effort by physicians to help their colleagues is the Washington State Medical Association's "Problem Doctor Rehabilitation Program."[3] Members of the association call on doctors whose practices are being affected by senility or other behavioral problems. They are not trying to "police" the profession, but to act early enough to afford the affected doctor a chance to rehabilitate himself. Similar programs are now in effect in other states.

Some factors involved in a case of senility from the standpoint of a state board are apparent in the following two examples:

Doctor B., a ninety-year old rural practitioner, was reported to the Virginia State Board of Medicine for overprescribing addictive drugs, particularly amphetamines. In one year, this doctor had purchased over 150,000 amphetamine tablets from a single pharmaceutical company and similar quantities from three or four other firms. When the board learned of these massive orders, it scheduled a three-man informal conference with Doctor B. At this meeting, also attended by the doctor's attorney, it was evident that the aged physician was undergoing senile changes. The conference lasted about three hours, with no resolution of the problem. The discussion revealed that Doctor B. was selling "pep pills" to anyone who asked for them at his office, but is was apparent that he was not aware of the gravity of his actions. It was also learned that on several occasions teenagers had looted his office to obtain drugs from his large cache. Doctor B. had reacted to these robberies by arming himself with a shotgun, which made people in his community fear that he might harm someone or himself.

At the end of the conference, Doctor B. said he would discontinue dispensing amphetamines. However, he did, in fact, continue to sell drugs to teenagers, truck drivers, and anyone else who wanted them. The board, therefore, had no alternative other than to convene a formal hearing, at which Doctor B. did not appear. His license to practice was revoked and, although the license was returned to the board's office, Doctor B. continued to practice and to sell pills. Three months after the revocation, a warrant was issued and his office searched. Doctor B. admitted seeing patients and dispensing drugs illegally, trying to justify his actions on the basis of his being the only physician in the community and that he was badly needed. He also pleaded poor health due to aortic surgery and the loss of an eye. The board issued an arrest warrant but before it could be served, Doctor B. died of natural causes at the age of 93.

This case illustrates some difficulties and complexities that may attend such situations. In seeking an equitable solution, the board had to deal with legal procedures which were both time-consuming and costly. A simpler solution would have been to place the offending physician in a nursing home or under some kind of supervisory care. While resolution of the problem may seem obvious, its accomplishment by way of the board's procedural approach might have presented difficulties.

A second example demonstrates that, in some instances at least, a similar problem can be resolved more readily:

Doctor S. was brought to the attention of the Virginia State Board of Medicine by members of his medical society who were concerned that his physical condition would prevent his caring for his patient properly. The board was informed that Doctor S.'s hospital privileges had already been curtailed. After a three-man informal conference at which Doctor S. was present, the board advised him to retire. When his initial reaction was negative, the board invoked the "Sick Doctor Act,"[4] which required that Doctor S. undergo a complete physical and mental examination. Results of the examination, along with the urgings of his personal physician, convinced Doctor S. to retire from active practice. He did retire in a dignified fashion and was honored by his community for his services to it.

The Virginia State Board of Medicine has had limited experience with cases involving physical disability. Physical disability, per se, apparently seldom requires retirement. Rather, physical impairment often leads to secondary mental or emotional disturbances or to drug problems, which become the primary cause of disability. Cases of this type are usually managed by the board's Psychiatric Advisory Committee. In the late 1940s, Alvarez[5, 6] described the syndrome of "little strokes" occurring in relatively young individuals and often leading to signs of errors in judgment on the part of those affected. The following example shows the sequence of events leading to an emotionally induced disability following organic brain damage:

Over a period of several years, when Doctor K. was in his early sixties, he began to show signs of decreasing capability, intellectual and memory defects, faulty judgment, etc. Although he tried to mask these lapses by an overconfident manner, friends, fellow physicians, and hospital personnel noticed his functional deficits. A report was made to the board, and the case was referred to the Psychiatric Advisory Committee, which recommended that Doctor K.'s license should not be renewed. Fortunately, Doctor K. had some insight into his problem; he agreed with the board's decision and retired from practice. In this case, early cerebral arteriosclerosis caused manifold personality changes and functional impairment.

Many state licensing laws provide for revocation of a license because of "unprofessional conduct." In Virginia the law has been amended to partially define unprofessional behavior, but in many states, it is left to the state medical board to establish the definition on a case-by-case basis.

Webster's[7] definition of "professional" includes the following: "characterized by or conforming to the technical or

ethical standards of a profession." The problem, then, becomes
to define ethical standards of the medical profession. A 1969
study[8] of state medical board disciplinary actions revealed that
during the preceding five years boards had taken 938 formal
actions, ranging from reprimands to revocations of licenses.
Behavioral factors which were often noted in these actions included improper behavior with a patient, irresponsible prescribing of drugs, tax evasion, illegal abortion (until recent
changes in abortion laws), fraud, and abuse.

In the category of "unprofessional behavior," Virginia law
includes the inability to practice medicine with skill and safety
due to illness, drunkenness, excessive use of drugs, narcotics, or
chemicals, or as the result of any mental or physical condition.[9]

Widespread change in societal patterns of living and standards of ethics inevitably influences attempts to define desirable
standards of professional behavior for the medical profession.
Remarkable technologic advances have further complicated
ethical issues and presented physicians with new dilemmas and
responsibilities. Such questions as the definition of life —
when it starts and when it ends — are controversial and, for
many physicians, threatening to their own professional and
personal philosophy. Changes in laws and consequent court
decisions have had great impact on medical practice. The 1973
U.S. Supreme Court decision on abortion,[10] the decision in the
Karen Quinlan case,[11] and a "death with dignity" law enacted
recently in California[12] are examples of legal changes. In the
face of all this, what criteria should a medical board — or, in
fact, any individual or group — follow to define unethical
behavior by a physician?

Another facet of the problem is that of advertising and the
commercialization of medical practice, with which the AMA
has been struggling for several years. In 1976, the Health Systems Agency of Northern Virginia successfully sued the Virginia State Board of Medicine to uphold a doctor's right to
limited advertising.[13] Certainly, few doctors would support the
use of blatant hucksterism, but questions of acceptable advertising are increasing and must be resolved.

The matter of incompetence must also be considered in any

discussion of unprofessional behavior. Several court cases have involved the question of whether incompetence constitutes unprofessional conduct. Although the answer seems obvious, strict interpretation of some state laws leaves room for doubt.

State licensing boards must deal with unprofessional, incompetent, unethical physicians, but their task is often not as relatively simple as the following example: Doctor G. had a large practice in a small Virginia community, with too many patients and too little time to handle them all. He began to delegate increasing responsibilities for patient care to an aide. Over a period of several years, the aide was seeing patients and dispensing medications while the doctor was out of the office. In this case, the board was able to resolve the problem with a strong written reprimand to the doctor.

This type of problem is becoming more acute because of the increasing use of allied health personnel such as physician's assistants and nurse practitioners. These individuals now perform acts once considered to be solely with the physician's province. Licensing boards must be concerned with the supervision physicians provide their assistants. The board must determine whether supervision is present and adequate or whether an assistant is, in fact, practicing medicine.

Although instances of alleged fraud and abuse are receiving much national publicity, verification of specific violations is difficult, and disciplinary action is not always feasible. Many elements are involved in such cases, including legal considerations. Defrauding Medicare/Medicaid programs is presently a misdemeanor, and legislation has been introduced to make it a felony.[14] It is vitally important, in dealing with complaints of fraud and abuse, for a state board to have access to all pertinent information and to have available the necessary legal expertise, as the following case demonstrates:

Doctor P., a young female physician, was first brought to the attention of the Virginia State Board of Medicine for alleged overbilling of third-party carriers. She was convicted of a felony, which in Virginia can result in an automatic suspension of license. Her license was suspended and she was referred to the medical board's Psychiatric Advisory Committee for evaluation. It was determined that Doctor P. had a number of emotional problems, resulting in some hostility from her toward the medical community. She was referred for private psychiatric care. Following treatment, her license was reinstated on a probationary status, but her professional conduct will be monitored indefinitely by the board.

Physicians are beginning to realize that as government intervention increases, there will be more scrutiny of their professional activities. Professional review sections have already been established for both the Medicare and Medicaid programs. These sections monitor and evaluate claims submitted by physician-providers to determine whether the claims are in line with the programs' provisions. Although Medicare-Medicaid systems have existed in the Commonwealth of Virginia since 1969, only in more recent years has significant action been taken to identify fraud and abuse. In the past two years, three Virginia practitioners have been convicted of fraud relative to Medicare/Medicaid and the CHAMPUS* program. Information from these agencies has led to three more cases now in the courts, and more investigations will be concluded in the near future.

Many practitioners involved in this type of fraud have claimed they were ignorant of the law or that they did not know of the alleged abuses because their clerical assistants filed the claims. No reminder is needed that ignorance of the law is not an acceptable plea and that the individual practitioner who signs the contract with the agencies is responsible for all claims. Even though a physician may not realize that clerical personnel are making mistakes on his claims, that physician is personally responsible for his employees' acts. Mistakes of this type may ultimately lead to a felony conviction and the loss of many personal rights. Physicians should conduct a bimonthly or quarterly review of all claims. If discrepancies are found, immediate notification to the agency concerned could save the physician both legal problems and personal embarrassment.

A difficult area to evaluate is that of patient complaints of

---

*Civilian Health and Medical Program of the Uniform Services.

improper advances or relationships. If true, such complaints fall into the category of unprofessional conduct. However, in many instances, they reflect a physician's underlying emotional or psychiatric problems. The Virginia State Board of Medicine has had very few convictions on this type of charge, and there have only been ten such formal complaints to the board in the last ten years. The small number can perhaps be explained by a patient's reluctance to pursue such a case with a formal complaint and testimony.

Often such complaints come from emotionally disturbed patients, but they still create problems for the physician. To avoid them, common sense should be the rule. For example, proper chaperons should always be present during complete examinations of female patients. A practitioner should recognize when a patient becomes disgruntled during an office visit and realize that patient may later make accusations concerning the physician's actions or comments. Fees should be discussed openly with the patient or family, preferably at the start of treatment. One should remember that once an accusation is made, even though it is later disproved, it is not easily forgotten. The public tends to remember the indictment rather than the exoneration, and doubt lingers. In most cases of this type handled by the Virginia board, complete patient satisfaction has never been attained.

Finally, a very "gray area" of board responsibility is that of the physician who, for whatever reason, maintains a drug addict. The Virginia law appears in the Virginia State Board of Pharmacy Regulations[15], and the applicable federal law is administered by the Drug Enforcement Administration[16]. Pertinent sections of the Virginia State Board of Pharmacy Regulations follow:

Regulation 16. Purpose of Issue of Prescriptions

A. A prescription for a controlled drug, in order to be valid, must be issued for a legitimate medical purpose by an individual practitioner acting in the usual course of his professional practice. The responsibility for the prescribing of controlled drugs, in good faith, is upon the prescribing practitioner, but a corresponding responsibility rests with the

pharmacist who fills the prescription. An order purporting to
be a prescription issued not in the usual course of professional treatment or in legitimate and authorized research is
not a prescription within the meaning and intent of Sections
54-524.65 and 54-524.66, and the person filling such a pur-
ported prescription knowingly, as well as the person issuing
it, shall be subject to the penalties provided for violation of
the provisions of law relating to controlled drugs.

B. An order issued by a practitioner to obtain controlled
drugs for the purpose of general dispensing to patients shall
not be considered a valid prescription.

C. A prescription may not be issued for the dispensing of
drugs listed in any schedule, to a drug dependent person for
the purpose of continuing his dependence upon such drugs,
in the course of conducting an authorized clinical investigation in the development of an addict rehabilitation program.

Regulation 17. Dispensing of Drugs for Maintenance Purposes

The administering or dispensing directly (but not prescribing) the drugs listed in any schedule to a narcotic drug
dependent person for the purpose of continuing his dependence upon such drugs, in the course of conducting an authorized program shall be deemed to be within the meaning of
the term "in good faith" in Section 54-524.65 and Section 54-
524.66, Code of Virginia, provided that approval is obtained
prior to the initiation of such a program by submission of a
Notice of Claimed Investigational Exemption for a New Drug
to the Food and Drug Administration which will be reviewed
concurrently by the Food and Drug Administration for scientific merit and by the Drug Enforcement Administration and
the Board of Pharmacy for drug control requirements and
that the clinical investigation thereafter accords with such
approval as required by Federal Regulations or by any Commonwealth Regulation of the Board of Pharmacy or the
Board of Medicine.

The intent of the law is clear: It is against the law to maintain
an addict by prescribing his drugs.

The Virginia board has encountered cases of a physician's
"treating" a member of his family, when, in reality, the physician and/or his wife was addicted. This type of situation is
nearly always brought to the board's attention by the Virginia
State Board of Pharmacy or by another physician. In such a

case, the first action taken is always a meeting with the physician himself. In nearly every instance in the Virginia board's experience, if the physician is maintaining an addict within his family, he is probably also addicted. In fact, he may be trying to justify his own addiction in terms of "treatment" of a family member who is "ill."

A related type of case is that of the terminally ill addict. This patient may already be addicted when first seen by a physician or, because of severe pain, may become addicted while under treatment. The classic example, of course, is the patient with severe pain from long-term neoplastic disease. The law allows a physician to *dispense*, but not prescribe, narcotics to a patient "in good faith," if, in his medical judgment, continued addiction is necessary.

In cases like this, the Virginia board often tries to persuade a physician to have his patient hospitalized, rather than to maintain the addiction. If this is not possible, the physician writes a letter to the board to be placed on file. The Virginia State Board of Pharmacy and the Drug Enforcement Administration are informed. The physician is instructed to fill his prescriptions for addictive drugs at one pharmacy, if possible, and he is monitored and allowed to continue administering the drugs. This is the exceptional case, rather than the rule, because there is no question that maintenance of an addict is against the law. Physician board members, however, must not lose sight of the fact that the practice of medicine is still an art — not all science — and that decisions "in good faith" are still in order.

The reputation of the medical profession has suffered in recent years. The reasons are varied, but physicians' behavior is certainly a factor. Cases of senility, incompetence, and unprofessional conduct, including fraud and abuse, must be reported to state boards, and the boards must deal with them effectively. If high standards of professionalism are to be upheld, the first step must be a high degree of exemplary professional behavior on the part of every practicing physician.

REFERENCES

1. AMA Committee on Aging: *Retirement: A Medical Philosophy and Approach.* N.D.

2. Duffy, J. C.: *Emotional Issues in the Lives of Physicians.* Springfield, Ill., Charles C Thomas Publisher, 71, 1970.
3. *AMA News:* December 20/27, 1976.
4. Commonwealth of Virginia. LAWS OF VIRGINIA RELATING TO MEDICINE AND OTHER HEALING ARTS. V, Sec. 54-317(11).
5. Alvarez, W. A.: Small commonly unrecognized strokes. *Postgrad Med, 4*:96-101, 1948.
6. _____: Cerebral arteriosclerosis with small commonly unrecognized apoplexies. *Geriatrics, 1*:189-216, 1946.
7. *Webster's New Collegiate Dictionary.* Springfield, Ma., G & C Merriam Company, 919, 1975.
8. Derbyshire, R. C.: Medical ethics and discipline. *JAMA, 228*:59-62, 1974.
9. Commonwealth of Virginia. LAWS OF VIRGINIA RELATING TO MEDICINE AND OTHER HEALING ARTS. V, Sec. 54-317.
10. Roe vs Wade, 93 Sup. Ct. 705, Jan. 22, 1973.
11. In the Matter of Karen Ann Quinlan, 355 Atlantic II 647 N.J. Super. Ct., Mar. 31, 1976.
12. CALIFORNIA HEALTH AND SAFETY CODE, Pt. 1, Div. VII 3.9 Sec. 718.5, Jan. 1, 1977.
13. Virginia Health Systems Agency of Northern Virginia, *et al.* vs Virginia State Board of Medicine, *et al.,* Di Ct. E.D.Va., 424 F. Supp. 267, Nov. 4, 1976.
14. Medicare-Medicaid Anti-Fraud and Abuse Amendments. H. R. 3, S. 143, Ninety-fifth Congress, First Session, Jan. 4, 1977 and Jan. 11, 1977.
15. Commonwealth of Virginia, BOARD OF PHARMACY REGULATIONS, 16, 17, Jan. 21, 1975.
16. Title 21, U.S. Code Fed. Reg. (CFR) 1306.04, 1306.07.

___Chapter 7___

LEGAL RIGHTS OF THE SICK
OR INCOMPETENT PHYSICIAN

$$\overline{}$$

BEFORE the late nineteenth century, the practice of medicine in the United States was virtually unregulated. The physician occupied a position of public trust and confidence unequaled by that of any other professional person. As American society became more urbanized and more sophisticated, the community of physicians developed from a rather dispersed population of general practitioners, with little or no organized hospital facilities, to a more centralized gathering of specialists in satellite groups around or in the highly technical facility known as the modern hospital. At the same time, the problem of the physician who, for various reasons, became incompetent or whose skills were impaired by illness or abuse of drugs grew increasingly acute.

Formerly, an impaired physician could continue to practice because there were no qualified peers in his community to detect his impairment or because he was able to conceal his impairment successfully. When impairment was obvious, as in some instances of alcoholism, the community may have lacked an acceptable alternative to the affected physician. Today, however, the situation is different. Both the public and the medical community have become more sophisticated and more insistent on quality health care delivery. Also, the public is now more critical of the medical profession and its ancillary disciplines. As a result, the practice of medicine and the other healing arts has become the object of increasing governmental regulation on both the national and state levels.

Until recently, the federal government has been content to leave professional regulatory matters to the individual states. However, with the advent of critical and organized consumer reaction to the "malpractice crisis," the U.S. Congress has begun to examine the problems of medical competence and

65

discipline. A possible result is the enactment of uniform federal standards, which could supersede or greatly modify the states' power to regulate the practice of medicine and allied professions. Whether this trend will continue and what its future impact will be upon the legal rights and duties of physicians and ancillary personnel remain to be seen. However, for the time being, the legal framework for regulating medical practice and the other healing arts is whatever the individual states have developed.

Every state has establishd some type of legislative formula to regulate the practice of medicine. These statutes are usually known as "Medical Practice Acts," or similar titles and set forth specific educational requirements for licensure for physicians and other practitioners of the healing arts and delineate conditions under which a license to practice may be revoked, suspended, or otherwise limited. Commonly, the administration of Medical Practice Acts has been vested in a medical board or commission. Usually, but not always, board members are physicians or practitioners of those other professions regulated. The board or commission functions as an administrative agency of the executive branch of the state government. The legislature has delegated to these boards or commissions the power to investigate practitioners suspected of breaches of discipline, to administratively adjudicate or try such cases, and, upon proof of charges, to remove or limit the license to practice.

In recent years, several states have recognized the unique problems posed by sick or incompetent physicians, and they have attempted to solve these problems by modifying existing regulatory mechanisms. In most cases, however, the sick or incompetent physician has not breached existing disciplinary rules or statutes which had been developed to deal with the dishonest or unethical practitioner. Therefore, the states have had to define a new category of prohibited or proscribed conduct and, for the most part, to establish new procedures for dealing with this new category of the sick or incompetent physician. Some states have also established standards for continuing medical education, with penalties for failure to comply, in order to cope with the professionally incompetent physician.

"Sick Doctor Acts" have been passed to identify and regulate practitioners whose ability to practice with safety to the public has been diminished. These acts usually provide that if there is probable cause to believe that a practitioner's ability has become so impaired that he poses a potential danger to his patients, after a preliminary investigation or an investigatory hearing, the regulatory board may direct the practitioner to undergo physical or psychiatric testing and treatment, with specific penalties for failure to comply. Subsequent to such testing or treatment, and after a full hearing, the regulatory board may impose appropriate restrictions on the practitioner's right to practice.[1]

Although the states have developed varying legislative restraints to cope with the physician who has breached a disciplinary rule or statute, and some states now have statutory procedures to deal with the sick or incompetent practitioner, a further question remains. What legal recourse does a practitioner have against any arbitrary or improper exercise of the regulatory power vested in state boards of medicine and related fields?

First, the right of a physician or practitioner of the other healing arts to practice his profession has been held to be a very valuable property right.[2] Accordingly, that property right is protected by the "due process" clause of the fourteenth amendment of the U.S. Constitution. The pertinent part states: "No state shall . . . deprive any person of life, liberty or property without due process of law." The "due process" clause and its interpretation over the years by both state and federal judiciary have come to be the primary bulwark of protection for the practitioner's right to practice his profession without undue arbitrary or improper interference by state regulatory boards.

As a result, Medical Practice Arts must conform to certain constitutional criteria evolving from the fourteenth amendment to the U.S. Constitution. The purpose of such acts is to protect the public from delivery of inadequate medical care by dishonest, incompetent, or sick physicians.[3] If the provisions of the acts are reasonable in relation to this purpose, those provisions will pass the constitutional test of the "due process" clause.[4] In this context, it is likely that as long as Sick Doctor Acts are reasonably specific regarding the conduct they are intended to prevent and are procedurally sound as to the means for accomplishing those ends, they will pass constitutional muster.

Since most professional regulatory boards are administrative agencies, functioning as part of the executive branch of government, the nature of those boards and the procedures by which they function should be examined. The principal duty of an administrative agency such as a board of medicine is to administer the laws — the Medical Practice Acts — that created the board in the first place. To administer these laws, the legislatures have delegated to the agencies concerned additional functions that are essentially legislative and judicial in nature. An administrative agency may supplement its basic law with regulations that are within the scope of its delegated authority, thus functioning as a quasi-legislative body. In addition, an administrative agency may investigate and adjudicate alleged violations of its disciplinary statutes or regulations. The fact that a medical board investigates, brings charges, and then proceeds to try the issues does not constitutionally disqualify the board's actions.[5]

Procedurally, the actions of medical boards in adjudicating issues involving violations of disciplinary statutes or regulations need not be as formal as the actions required by the criminal adjudicative process. Standards of proof and other evidential considerations are considerably less rigid in administrative proceedings because of their essentially civil, as opposed to criminal, nature.[6] The United States Supreme Court has held that the "due process" clause of the U.S. Constitution does not require any particular formal procedure in administrative adjudications. However, the accused must be granted reasonable notice of the proceedings and the charges against him, and he must be afforded a reasonable opportunity to present defense.[7] If these two fundamental requirements — notice and the opportunity to be heard — are not met, the fundamental fairness requirement of the "due proess" clause is violated, and the administrative action will be negated. Some notice requirements imposed by the courts are that the accused be personally notified of the charges and pending proceedings[8] and that the specification of charges or complaints delivered to the accused be sufficiently precise to allow him to prepare his defense.[9] The hearing must be fair in appearance as well as in form and substance,[10] but it need not be controlled by criminal law procedural rules or precedents.[11] An important distinction is that administrative hearings need not be bound by results of prior related criminal proceedings. Administrative boards may make their own independent findings of fact from evidence adduced at their own hearings.[12]

Most, if not all, states have codified court decisions requiring certain procedural safeguards in either the Medical Practice Acts themselves or in the states' Administrative Procedure Acts.[13] Included are the accused's right to present witnesses in his own behalf and to be allowed some limited prehearing examination of the evidence to be presented against him. Another aspect of administrative adjudicatory proceedings, which warrants special mention, is the standard of evidence which reviewing courts have uniformly held to be sufficient to support an administrative board's order. It has been held consistently that a reviewing court may not disturb a board's order if it is apparent from the record of the board proceedings that the order is supported by "substantial evidence." The quantum of evidence required to meet the "substantial evidence" test is difficult to assess, since it depends on the facts and circumstances of each particular case. However, it is my judgment that most reviewing courts will not require the findings of an administrative tribunal to meet a standard of evidence higher than the "preponderance of the evidence" test of the civil courts. In criminal courts the standard is stricter, requiring "evidence beyond a reasonable doubt." Indeed, courts have even allowed more weight than would be indicated by the "preponderance" test to the findings of administrative agencies, such as medical boards, in view of their peculiar expertise.

Most Administrative Procedure Acts provide for judicial review of administrative agency actions.[14] Even in states that do not have specific Administrative Procedure Acts, the Medical

Practice Acts usually provide for some type of review by the courts upon appeal by the practitioner affected by a medical board order. Often the courts are closed to a practitioner who seeks judicial intervention in medical board proceedings, unless all required agency action is completed. This is the doctrine of exhaustion of administrative remedies. Another criterion for court review has been that of jurisdiction. Most, if not all states have provided their courts with jurisdiction over final agency actions either by virtue of the states' Administrative Procedure Acts or the basic law establishing the agencies. These statutes provide the courts with guidelines for the scope of a review as well as the permissible court action upon completion of the review. One significant factor, however, that results from the constitutional doctrine of separation of executive, legislative, and judicial powers, is that the courts' power to review decisions of administrative agencies applies only to the agencies' *exercise* of their statutory powers, and not to the *merits* of the decisions reached by the agencies. Therefore, the courts will not reverse agency actions unless there has been a clear abuse of the agency's discretion as vested in it by the legislature.[15]

In the past, the federal courts have refused to intervene in state administrative proceedings.[16] More recently, there has been a trend for the federal district courts to use the Civil Rights Act of 1964[17] as a vehicle to scrutinize certain aspects of state administrative agency actions. One aspect that merits special mention relates to recent federal court cases that have attacked the composition of certain state regulatory boards as to their potential for bias or prejudice as it affects their capacity to adjudicate cases. A case of note involved the Alabama Board of Optometry whose membership was by law limited to the members of the state professional optometric association. The professional association excluded those optometrists who were associated with large commercial firms. The board had, in fact, promulgated regulations which severely restricted the right of those commercial optometrists to practice their profession. When the board instituted proceedings against those optometrists, they repaired to the federal courts.

The U.S. Supreme Court struck down the Alabama Board's

actions by holding that the board's composition was tainted with bias and that such patently unfair action by the board was constitutionally impermissible.[18] Other federal cases have extended the potential for bias into areas of strictly economic consideration.[19]

In order to counter such decisions, some states have passed statutes mandating the use of administrative hearing officers or examiners to preside over agency adjudications. Such hearing officers are not associated with the agency for which they preside and are usually given broad powers to find facts, reach conclusions of law, and, in some cases, propose sanctions. The agency is usually limited to reviewing the actions of the hearing officer. Such a system has worked well in the state of Virginia and should offset some of the far-reaching aspects of federal court decisions.

Formal actions by medical boards are usually the most drastic actions that will confront the sick or incompetent physician. In most cases, it is believed that the boards, remembering that their basic purpose is not to punish a practitioner but to protect the public, will use the least restrictive procedures possible in order to rehabilitate the sick or incompetent physician and return him to a useful role in the delivery of health care.

REFERENCES

1. See, for instance, Sec. 54-317(11) of the CODE OF VIRGINIA (1950), *as amended,* which reads in pertinent part as follows: "Any practitioner of medicine . . . shall be considered guilty of unprofessional conduct if he: (") . . . is unable to practice medicine with reasonable skill and safety to patients by reason of illness, drunkeness, etc."
2. Korndorffer vs Texas State Board of Medical Examiners, 460 S.W. 2d 879 (Tex 1970); Hughes vs State Board of Medical Examiners, 162 Ga. 246, 134 S.E. 42 (1926).
3. Young vs State Board of Registration for the Healing Arts, 451 S.W. 2d 346 (Mo. 1969); Yakov vs Board of Medical Examiners, 68 Cal. 2d 67, 435 P. 2d 553 (1968).
4. Meffert vs The State Board of Medical Registration and Education, 66 Kan. 710, 72 P. 247 (1903).
5. Larkin vs Withrow, 421 U.S. 132, 95 Sup. Ct. 1456 (1974); Seidenberg vs New Mexico Board of Medical Examiners, 452 P. 2d 469 (N.M. 1969).

6. Margoles vs Wisconsin State Board of Medical Examiners, 177 N.W. 2d 353 (Wisc. 1970).
7. State of Missouri *ex rel* Hurwitz vs North, *et al.,* Board of Health of the State of Missouri, 271 U.S. 40; 46 S.Ct. 384 (1925).
8. Bruni vs Department of Registration and Education of the State of Illinois, 290 N.E. 2d 295 (Ill. 1972).
9. Kansas Board of Healing Arts vs Foote. 436 P. 2d 828 (Kan. 1968).
10. Campbell vs Board of Medical Examiners, 518 P. 2d 1042 (Ore. Ct. Appeals, 1974).
11. Shakin vs Board of Medical Examiners, 487 Cal. Rptr. 274 (Cal. Ct. App. 1967).
12. Young vs State Board of Registration for the Healing Arts, 451 S.W. 2d 346 (Mo. 1969).
13. See, for instance, Sec. 9-6.14:10 through 9-6.14:14 of the CODE OF VIRGINIA (1950), *as amended.* (The Administrative Process Act, Article 3, *Case Decisions*).
14. See, for instance, Sec. 9-6.14:15 through 9-6.14:19 of the CODE OF VIRGINIA (1950), *as amended.* (The Administrative Process Act, Article 4, *Court Review*).
15. *Ibid.*[5]
16. Geiger vs Jenkins, 316 F. Supp. 370 (D.C.Ga. 1970); Prosch vs Baxley, 345 F. Supp. 1063 (D.C. Ala. 1973).
17. 42 U.S.C.A. 1981 *et seq.*
18. Gibson vs Berryhill, 411 U.S. 564, 93 S. Ct. 1689.
19. Wall vs American Optometric Association, *et al.,* 379 F. Supp. 175 (N.D. Ga. 1974 *affirmed* U.S.Sup. Ct. October 21, 1974). *Justice vs Georgia State Board of Examiners in Optometry* (Companion case to *Wall*).

Chapter 8

THE MEDICAL PROFESSION'S RESPONSIBILITY TOWARD THE IMPAIRED PHYSICIAN

THE medical profession has much of which to be proud. Its history abounds with a long list of magnificent clinical achievements; it maintains high ethical standards, and it provides superior educational and training programs. Yet, in spite of these credits, it is indisputable — and saddening — that the profession has largely failed in its responsibility toward its own impaired and incompetent members. Evidence of this failure was presented in a 1961 AMA study[1] on professional discipline, which stressed that apathy, ignorance, and a lack of responsibility by physicians generally existed in regard to the impaired and incompetent physician.

Since that report, responsible members of organized medical groups and state medical boards have made a strenuous effort to provide guidelines and regulations that the profession can use in its efforts to establish adequate self-discipline. Despite these herculean efforts by a few, there has been very little change in the average physician's attitude toward more effective professional discipline. Why does this apathy exist? Why is there still so much obvious evidence of incompetence and gross deviant behavior within the profession? Why do members of the profession do so little about these deviant physicians?

Too often, it is only after flagrant evidence of personality disruption or a blatant instance of incompetence, which the press has probably exposed, that local and state medical disciplinary bodies appear to recognize the problem and take action. Why are such problem physicians not detected earlier in the course of their mental or physical illness? Why are they allowed to continue their deviant behavior patterns until a disaster occurs?

Obviously, the answers to such questions are complex and involve a multitude of variables. In the discussion that follows we attempt to define more clearly the profession's responsibility toward its impaired members and to delineate many of the factors involved in failure either to recognize or to act appropriately when problems occur.

The manifestation of deviant behavior is often insidious. Common causes of incompetence include alcohol and drug abuse, mental illness, senility, and professional obsolescence. Early signs of these problems are usually subtle and not easily detected. Often a physician with one or a combination of these problems may practice alone and may be able to maintain acceptable patient records. Because no other physician directly monitors the patients clinically, the impaired physician may conceal his disability or incompetence and cover his failures by medical transfers, early hospital discharges, or poor documentation. It is more difficult to recognize the problem if such physicians do not practice in a hospital. In this solitary situation any peer surveillance is almost impossible. The impaired physician's downhill path will continue until some disastrous event brings him to the attention of his peers or of local authorities.

Even when common signs and symptoms of incompetence become moderately advanced, recognition or action may still be difficult. It is all too common that one watches a colleague drink excessively at parties for many years. When does one realize that this physician has lost control and that his drinking has begun to limit his judgment and impair his performance? Should action be taken when it becomes known he has been stopped in his car by the local police and taken home, without being ticketed for drunken driving? Should disciplinary action be taken when the nursing "grapevine" reports that often when this physician is called during the night, he does not answer but, instead, his wife says he is "too ill" to talk? Yet, the next day he appears at work, presumably able to function. How long should peers and, indeed, friends wait for further evidence of deteriorating behavior before acknowledging that such a colleague is significantly impaired?

The problem of recognition is also difficult with physicians who become addicted to drugs. This form of deviant behavior has equally subtle signs. Frequently, it occurs among the most successful and dedicated of our colleagues. Since most physicians seldom think of self-administration of drugs as a problem for either themselves or their colleagues, such a manifestation of aberrant behavior usually occurs over a long period before it is recognized. Too often, it is the disappearance of narcotics from hospital stores, patently inappropriate behavior, or the discovery by a state pharmacy inspector of fraudulent prescriptions that leads to disclosure of the situation. By the time this happens, however, the addiction is advanced, and the affected physician's clinical competence has become inadequate.

Probably the most difficult problem to recognize is senility in the aging physician. Even physicians of great ability often lapse so subtly into this aging process that only minimal manifestations are evident at an early stage. Long-standing skills often mask faulty performance, and colleagues are surprised when inappropriate responses to clinical problems finally become apparent. The physician in solo practice who becomes senile may do inestimable harm before other problems of aging take their toll, or before his records and clinical work clearly indicate his incompetence.

Physical disability may be simpler to recognize since it is usually more obvious to all observers. Such entities as severe angina, progressive emphysema, degenerative arthritis, parkinsonism, or the residual physical effects of a cerebral vascular accident frequently affect older physicians, decreasing their ability to function capably.

Although problems of physical disability are the easiest to recognize, they are perhaps the most difficult to manage because they do not stem from self-indulgence, and the afflicted physician's mental faculties may be unaffected.

Mental illness, excluding that caused by drugs or alcohol, is seldom detected in colleagues at an early stage. Depression, one of the more common problems, often goes unrecognized until it culminates in complete deterioration of performance and neglect of clinical responsibility, or in suicide. Other forms of mental illness also affect the physician population but, even when recognized, colleagues seldom take any action.

The fact that recognition of deviant behavior is sometimes difficult does not excuse the failure of the profession to take responsible action. Too often many types of incompetence are recognized, but little is done. Why is there a lack of motivation to become involved in the unpleasantness of disciplinary action? The philosophies of "live and let live" and "there but for the Grace of God go I" are some excuses for inaction. In addition, lifelong friendships or loss of referral sources may be factors deterring an individual physician from initiating or taking part in disciplinary actions.

Other determinant factors, too, are involved once incompetence or deviant behavior is recognized, even in early stages. Many physicians and hospital staffs have great difficulty defining incompetence and do not know how to document it. The criteria of competence are admittedly vague. The definition used earlier suggests that competence is good medical practice according to accepted current methods. The difficulties of interpreting this definition are obvious, particularly if disciplinary procedures are likely to be challenged and ultimately taken to court. We can all recognize and define gross patterns of poor practice, but it is much harder to define, document, and ultimately prove less dramatic inadequacies.

One of the major obstacles to successful disciplinary action against physicians has been the inadequacy of hospital staff bylaws. Many such articles are antiquated, do not provide an adequate framework for disciplinary action, and seldom provide mechanisms for appeal or redress by the accused physician. Even the most highly motivated physician understandably becomes frustrated and defeated when there is little support or guidance from staff bylaws to instigate disciplinary procedures against an incompetent colleague. Within the legalistic framework of todays world, few physicians are willing to challenge a colleague who may become hostile and vindictive, unless there is assurance that institutional bylaws are well conceived, up-to-date, and can serve as a specific guide for this difficult undertaking.

The Joint Commission on Accreditation of Hospitals (JCAH) has been advocating the modernization of hospital bylaws. The JCAH has provided a step-by-step plan for disciplinary procedures along with a parallel appeal mechanism to ensure the rights of an accused physician.[2] Despite these well-laid-out plans, most hospital staff members still feel awkward in attempting to deal with an obviously incompetent physician who has not committed an act for which he can formally be judged incompetent. This situation has been the despair of many conscientious hospital staff members, and it has often resulted in much adverse publicity for the profession. Fortunately, with the advent of the Florida Sick Doctor Statute[3] as a model, the problem can be resolved. It is not legally possible for staff bylaws to include provisions for questioning a physician's fitness to practice medicine before his clinical judgment and skills become openly impaired. It is also possible to require medical and psychiatric evaluations of physicians whose behavior and actions are abnormal and to prevent the kind of personal and professional tragedies that have so often shamed and embarrassed the profession, or harmed patients.

Experience is another factor that enters into professional policing. Even with the most advanced guidelines, medical disciplinary committees often do not recognize the severity of an accused physician's problem or know what disciplinary action should be taken. An unfortunate common occurrence is the appointment of inexperienced physicians to disciplinary committees where they tend to handle serious disciplinary problems poorly. Only after many years of repeated exposure to such problems do physicians seem to reach a truly effective level of performance. Since most appointments to disciplinary committees are rotated among hospital staff members, it is quite difficult for the committees to maintain an effective level of experience. Further, disciplinary procedures are inherently highly charged emotionally and take a tremendous toll in time and mental stress. Many physicians are simply not able to cope adequately with problems of this nature, and they should not be forced into hearings and confrontations for which their temperaments and personalities are unsuited. Hospital staffs would do well to recognize those physicians who are capable of doing an effective job and keep them on disciplinary committees as long as they will serve effectively.

Paralleling the problem of intrahospital disciplinary procedures is the difficulty that local and state medical societies have in handling the deviant physician. In cases involving physicians without hospital affiliation, or cases not handled by hospital staffs, there have often been no organizations empowered to act other than state medical boards. Unfortunately, local and state medical societies are poorly equipped to administer meaningful discipline because their powers are usually limited to withdrawing membership privileges and expressing peer disapproval.

The public finds it extremely difficult to understand the inability of medical societies to be more effective in policing their own ranks. This lack of effective means of disciplinary action, although due in part to the varying nature of medical societies, does not excuse these groups. Many such organizations have obviously avoided responsible disciplinary action whenever possible and, because of inertia, poor organization, and indifference, have ignored or inadequately investigated the most flagrant violations of professional competence. Until these societies make a concerted effort to acknowledge their responsibilities for effectively disciplining their members, the public will continue to show increasing disenchantment with the profession's efforts at self-discipline.

Fortunately, some state medical societies are now involving themselves in the investigative and disciplinary functions of their state boards and are developing mechanisms for voluntary reporting of physical or mental incompetence and for instigating appropriate treatment. This is a positive approach which should become standard practice in every state. The manpower needed for adequate investigation of the many professional problems requiring attention is not available at either the medical society or state board level. But a combination of state board and state medical society members, acting in concert, promises to be a major factor in more effectively dealing with incompetent physicians and thereby helping to restore public confidence in the medical profession.

State medical boards have not been beyond criticism in their handling of sick and impaired physicians. Traditionally, these boards have been considered the sole professional organizations equipped by law and experience to deal most effectively with sick and incompetent physicians. However, many boards have done a very limited and ineffectual job. National summaries of board actions, license revocations, and probations indicate an appalling lack of action[4, 5] until recently. Here again, a partial excuse has been the difficulty in working within the framework of state medical acts coupled with a reluctance to revoke a physician's license and thus take away his livelihood.

No plan of professional self-discipline can be successful without adequate laws to require the reporting of sick and incompetent physicians to state medical boards. It is our belief that such state laws should require health-care institutions to report officially any physician who is found to be medically incompetent or medically unable to practice medicine. Further, we believe that any physician who is either voluntarily or involuntarily hospitalized for drug addiction, chronic alcoholism, or disabling psychiatric reasons should similarly be reported to his state board of medicine. Such reporting would not necessarily be for punitive or disciplinary action but would allow the board to monitor the physician's activities and to ensure that adequate treatment is provided and that rehabilitation is successful. Such a law has been enacted in Virginia and includes immunity for those reporting and adequate confidentiality for those reported.[7]*

The absence of such laws in most states permits an environment which allows chronically ill and incompetent physicians to continue to care for an unsuspecting public. Many physicians have repeated hospitalizations or commitments for drug addiction, alcoholism, or psychiatric reasons. Yet, neither their peers nor hospital disciplinary committees are officially aware of their problems. Therefore, it is absolutely necessary that state

---

*Parts of this law now appear to be in conflict with federal law and regulations dealing with the confidentiality of alcohol and drug patient records. However fifteen states have enacted legislation making the reporting of medical malpractice mandatory.

medical societies and state boards of medicine recognize the problem and encourage their state legislatures to provide adequate laws to ensure regular reporting of cases which require investigation and remedial action.

The profession has been allowed self-government which does not originate in natural or constitutional rights. It is a privilege granted by the public which, in the past, has believed that it lacked the knowledge and expertise to review the quality of professional services and the ability to evaluate professional judgment. Should the public become increasingly concerned that its trust in the medical profession has not been honored, the privilege of self-management that medicine has enjoyed so long could well be severely restricted, and the public could become actively involved in regulating and policing the practicing physician.

Organized medicine has very little time left to rectify the damage caused by its past failures and apparent lack of interest in policing its own house. Clearly, the medical profession must reverse this situation or lose its traditional rights of self-management and a large segment of its self-esteem. The need for mechanisms to adequately monitor professional competence is now recognized. The essential goals are to instill in all physicians an awareness of their responsibility, to use current guidelines and laws effectively, and to develop new disciplinary means for the management of the sick and incompetent physician. Even more important is the need to alert the profession to the occupational hazards and common mental illnesses that all too often befall the practicing physician. Lack of recognition of these hazards and illnesses, particularly in their early stages, must be remedied by a concerted educational effort on the part of every medical organization. Not until the practicing physician is as alert to the illnesses that may affect himself and colleagues as he is to their occurrence in his patients will the problems of adequate physician self-management be resolved.

REFERENCES

1. Report of Medical Disciplinary Committee to the Board of Trustees.

American Medical Association, 52, June 1961.

2. Guidelines for the Formulation of Medical staff Bylaws, Rules and Regulations. Joint Commission on Accreditation of Hospitals, 18-30, 1971.

3. (a) Sec. 2, 69-205, LAWS OF FLORIDA; (b) FLORIDA STATUTE 458-1201 (1)(N); (a) is reference to Florida Medical Practice Act and (b) is "Sick Doctor Statute," passed in 1969 and added to (a).

4. Derbyshire, R. C.: *Medical Licensure and Discipline in the United States.* Baltimore, The Johns Hopkins Press, 7-79, 1969.

5. _____: Medical ethics and discipline. *JAMA, 228:*59-62, 1974.

6. AMA News Release: Summary sheet of national medical disciplinary actions, June 19, 1977, Chicago.

7. Committee Amendment in the nature of a substitute for House bill 1558, Virginia Assembly, 1977.

Chapter 9

THE VIRGINIA EXPERIENCE

THE effectiveness of state medical boards has frequently been questioned, in part because of their apparent unwillingness or inability to provide comprehensive statistics that would reflect their experiences in disciplining members of the medical profession. Only recently have any meaningful data been available to adequately assess state board disciplinary performance. These data are reflected in a summary of forty-seven state board actions from 1971 to 1976 provided by the AMA (Table 9-I).[1] It must be noted, however, that state boards operate under a maze of differing state medical codes which vary in effectiveness in regard to adequate authority to carry out disciplinary measures.

TABLE 9-I

SUMMARY OF DISCIPLINARY ACTIONS
FORTY-SEVEN STATE MEDICAL BOARDS*

	1971	1972	1973	1974	1975	1976
Disciplinary Actions Initiated	1,275	2,406	2,458	2,675	3,305	4,237
License Revocation	45	119	52	107	89	130
License revoked but stayed with probation	57	102	120	120	149	185
Narcotic Permit Suspension	28	32	43	71	93	121
Reprimand and Censure	26	27	43	66	101	163

*From AMA News Release, June 19, 1977, Chicago.

The State of Virginia's effectiveness in establishing disciplinary procedures for erring constituent physicians compares most favorably with that of the forty-six other states summarized in Table 9-I by the AMA. Indeed, when these national statistics are reduced to the average number of disciplinary procedures per state per year, Virginia's experience is impressive.

The Virginia experience is presented for the ten years 1967 to 1976 (Tables 9-II, 9-III and 9-IV), as it was during this period that significant advances were made in establishing the board's authority and disciplinary procedures and in maintaining adequate records. The cases reported in Tables 9-II and 9-III were reviewed and categorized individually. In those instances where multiple conditions existed, only the primary diagnosis was used. As indicated in these tables, the numbers refer only to newly reported cases and do not reflect the ongoing surveillance on which the board has frequently insisted.

Until 1967, the board's effectiveness had been limited by inadequate and ineffective regulations, a reluctance on the part of the profession to participate in disciplinary actions, and a certain innocence on the part of the public concerning its rights to protection from medical incompetence. During 1967, the Virginia State Board of Medicine, responding to an increasing demand from the public, the press, and the medical profession for more effective disciplinary procedures, encouraged the passage of new legislative acts, one of which provides for investigative powers in dealing with sick and incompetent physicians. This new authority made it possible for the first time for investigative teams, consisting of three board members, to require that physicians reported for infractions of the state medical code meet with the board's representatives in a nonjudicial setting. During these so-called informal conferences, disciplinary measures up to but not including revocation of licensure can be instituted. Although informality is encouraged, the accused physician may be represented by legal counsel. Should revocation of a license be recommended under this procedure it is necessary to have a full board hearing in a semijudicial setting, with proper legal representation for both the board and the accused physician.

Also in 1967, it became apparent to the board that some form of psychiatric guidance and evaluation was needed to deal with

TABLE 9-II

SUMMARY OF DISCIPLINARY ACTIVITIES
VIRGINIA STATE BOARD OF MEDICINE
1967 to 1976

	1967	1968	1969	1970	1971	1972	1973	1974	1975	1976	Totals
1. Revocation of License	6	3	2	5	7	5	3	10	11	7	59
2. License on Probation	16	9	9	13	9	7	22	15	31	25	156
3. Formal Hearings	0	0	0	0	0	2	4	4	4	5	18
4. Informal Hearings	0	2	4	0	2	1	17	10	8	7	51

5. Psychiatric Advisory Committee Cases	19	11	8	13	19	8	14	16	32	26	174
6. Board Hearings Only	3	0	2	3	5	7	4	4	8	1	37
7. Patient Complaints	0	0	0	1	2	5	10	15	16	25	74
Totals	44	25	25	35	44	35	74	74	110	96	569

TABLE 9-III

SUMMARY OF MEDICAL CODE VIOLATIONS
HANDLED BY THE
VIRGINIA STATE BOARD OF MEDICINE
1967 to 1976

	1967	1968	1969	1970	1971	1972	1973	1974	1975	1976	Totals
1. Drugs											
a. Physicians addicted	1	5	4	3	1	2	3	4	6	9	38
b. Indiscriminate prescribing/dispensing	1	6	2	6	4	7	22	13	7	8	76
c. Maintaining Addicts	1	0	0	1	1	0	2	0	5	3	13
d. Writing or dispensing for wife/husband	1	2	1	1	0	1	2	3	5	5	21
2. Alcohol	2	0	2	2	2	0	2	3	1	1	15
3. Psychiatric Illness	5	1	1	0	0	2	3	3	3	3	21

											Total
4. Senility	0	0	0	0	1	1	1	1	2	2	8
5. Incompetence/Malpractice (diagnosis/treatment not up to standard)	3	1	0	0	0	2	2	3	2	2	15
6. Unprofessional Conduct (disapproved personal relationship w/patients)	1	2	1	0	2	0	0	1	2	1	10
7. Fraud	3	0	0	0	0	0	0	2	1	1	7
8. Practicing Without A License	2	0	1	2	0	2	6	3	0	1	17
9. Other Violations	2	3	6	5	6	13	18	30	9	23	115

TABLE 9-IV

PHYSICIANS LICENSED AND
PRACTICING IN STATE OF VIRGINIA
1967 to 1976

1967	—	5,522
1968	—	4,660
1969	—	4,413
1970	—	5,307
1971	—	4,823
1972	—	5,191
1973	—	6,146
1974	—	6,882
1975	—	6,609
1976	—	7,038

the increasing number of physicians seen for problems related to alcohol, drugs, and mental illness. As a result, the board appointed a Psychiatric Advisory Committee, consisting initially of three independent psychiatrists, to conduct interviews, to evaluate this type of disciplinary problem, and to advise the board. From this beginning, a valuable system has evolved to provide continuing monitoring and advice concerning the treatment and rehabilitation of mentally ill physicians. At present, there are three teams of psychiatric advisors, each consisting of three psychiatrists, prudently located throughout the state, who meet with and advise the board.

In 1968, the board acknowledged its responsibility not only to maintain physician competence at the time of licensure but also throughout a practitioners professional career. Since then, the board has strongly advocated mandatory continuing education for relicensure to insure ongoing competence. Unfortunately, the Virginia State Medical Society has not accepted this concept. The result is that the state has no legal means of assuring continued competence after a medical license is issued.

During 1973, the board formed a closer working relationship with the Virginia State Board of Pharmacy. This cooperative effort and the diligence of the pharmacy inspectors have greatly increased the number of cases of drug abuse and addiction reported to the Virginia State Board of Medicine. Many of the board's current strong disciplinary actions stem from this program.

A further significant action in 1973 was the board's sponsorship of a legislative bill labelled, "The Sick Doctor Act." Passage of this bill by the state legislature allows the board to limit or revoke a physician's license if, after proper investigation, he is found to be mentally or physically incompetent. This has made it possible to restrict or terminate a physician's practice before rather than after he commits acts of incompetence. The bill states:[2]

> Any practitioner of medicine shall be considered guilty of unprofessional conduct if he conducts his practice in a manner contrary to the standards of ethics of his branch of the healing arts or in such a manner as to make his practice a danger to the health and welfare of his patient or to the public; or is unable to practice medicine with reasonable skill and safety to patients by reason of illness, drunkenness, excessive use of drugs, narcotics, chemicals or any other type of material or as a result of any mental or physical condition. In enforcing this subsection, the Board shall upon probable cause, and upon preliminary investigation by informal conference, have authority to compel a practitioner to submit to a mental or physical examination by physicians designated by it. Failure of a practitioner to submit to such examination when directed shall constitute an admission of the allegations against him, unless the failure was due to circumstances beyond his control, consequent upon which a default and final order may be entered without the taking of testimony or

presentation of evidence. A physician affected under this sub-section shall, at reasonable intervals, be afforded an opportunity to demonstrate that he can resume the competent practice of medicine with reasonable safety to patients;

In 1974, after the Virginia legislature passed a Freedom of Information Act, the board began publishing the names of physicians whose licenses had been placed on probation or revoked. These names appear in a quarterly newsletter circulated to the members of the Virginia medical profession. In 1976, the same information was sent to all hospitals granting privileges to physicians whose licenses were placed on probation or revoked.

In 1976, for the first time, the Board hired a full-time professional investigator to help gather evidence in cases reported for serious infractions of the medical code. Experience since then has indicated that several additional investigators could readily be utilized.

Much adverse criticism has been directed at state medical boards because of their alleged neglect of disciplinary procedures. In many cases this criticism may be justified. Yet it must be clearly understood that a state board of medicine may act only if physicians' disciplinary problems are reported to them. Further, after such reporting, there must be adequate laws to provide the boards with authority to investigate and to act. Unless these criteria are met, little effective action can be anticipated from medical disciplinary boards.

Virginia has been fortunate in that during the last decade an increasing number of effective controls and laws have evolved which have provided the Virginia State Board of Medicine with increasing authority.

One of the significant changes that have ensued since 1970 has been the public's increasing willingness to provide the board with specific complaints. Table 9-II clearly shows the rapid rise in consumer concern with various phases of medical care, starting with only one complaint in 1970 and thereafter increasing to a high of 74 in 1976. This represents an expanding awareness on the part of the public that it now has access to a concerned authority when confronted with adverse medical experiences. These increases in patient complaints also reflect an effort on the part of the Virginia State Board of Medicine to become more responsive to the public and to its problems with the profession. Obviously, not all of these complaints were found to be valid, but after investigation, many were found to be justified and led to disciplinary action.

There has been considerable adverse comment in the press and by some political figures about the limited number of licenses revoked by state medical boards throughout the country. Virginia's record of revoking fifty-nine licenses in the past ten years is not one in which the board takes pride (Table 9-II). The revocation of a medical license represents not only the board's failure to find a satisfactory rehabilitation plan, but also a personal and professional tragedy for the physician involved.

That 156 licenses have been placed on probation is probably a better reflection of effective action than is licensure revocation, because most medical code infractions do not warrant licensure revocation as much as discipline combined with rehabilitation. Probation is always combined with stipulations and limitations and is not, as many imply, a wrist-slapping procedure devoid of significant disciplinary impact. It is significant that there was a marked increase in the number of physicians placed on probation from 1967 through 1976, with a major increase starting in 1973. This reflects greater cooperation of the Virginia State Board of Pharmacy as well as passage of the "Virginia Sick Doctor Act." In 1967, a disproportionate number of licenses were placed on probation; this reflected the establishment of an informal investigating committee of the board as well as the establishment of the Psychiatric Advisory Committee.

Through the mechanism of "informal" hearings, the three-man committee of board members investigating a case often recommended revocation of licensure. Since the committee's disciplinary authority did not include licensure revocation, "formal" hearings were necessary during which the entire fourteen-member board and the accused physician, both represented by legal counsel, would meet. Such formal hearings were semijudicial and allowed the accused physician adequate legal defense and redress. The frequency of these hearings is also noted in Table 9-II. Since 1974, changes in the legislative code have made it possible for a "hearing officer," who must be a lawyer appointed by the Virginia State Supreme Court, to preside over the formal hearings without the presence of the full board. The decisions of the hearing officer are binding on the board. As a technical matter of law, and only after discovery of an error in the record, can the board reverse such a decision. Despite the absence of a medical background, the hearing officers perform well and their decisions are seldom challenged.

Still another form of disciplinary procedure, not previously described, is the "board hearing." At these hearings, physicians are interviewed by the entire fourteen-member board for a variety of reasons, including appeals against probation as well as violations of probation (Table 9-II). Licenses may not be revoked during these board hearings.

It has been noted that since 1973 the Virginia State Board of Medicine has been working closely with inspectors of the Virginia State Board of Pharmacy, and this effort is reflected in an increasing number of physicians apprehended for drug addiction and related drug offenses (Table 9-III).

The number of drug-addicted physicians reported to the board is of great concern. Since 1973, there has been a gradual increase in this figure, with a record of nine in 1976 (Table 9-III). With improved case findings, the board expects the number of drug-addicted physicians reported to continue to increase.

The high incidence of physicians dispensing narcotics to their wives is a significant corollary to drug addiction among physicians, while the maintenance of physician addicts by other physicians is often symptomatic of ignorance, bad judgment, and, at times, a self-serving motivation (Table 9-III).

Of special interest is the significant decrease in indiscriminate dispensing and prescribing by physicians (Table 9-III). Such practices consist largely of dispensing drugs without a proper physician-patient relationship. The decreased number of these offenses reported since a high of twenty-two in 1973, at least in part, may be due to the board's firm disciplinary posture and its public consequences.

The low incidence of physicians seen for alcoholism by the board is of concern and reflects the profession's wide acceptance of chronic alcoholism among its members. Between 1967 and 1976 the board reviewed only fifteen cases of alcoholism, with little change in the number of cases reported annually in recent years (Table 9-III). It has been said that 6 to 10 percent of all physicians who drink will become chronic alcoholics.[3] If this is a true estimate of alcoholism in the profession, it certainly has not been confirmed by the number of Virginia physicians reported to our board. We feel that chronic alcoholism in the medical profession is not receiving the attention, reporting, and disciplinary action that is needed, and that the blame must rest with local hospital staffs and medical societies for continuing to tolerate this problem.

Disabling psychiatric illness represents a different kind of disciplinary problem. During the past ten years, the board has investigated twenty-one such cases, of which eight involved physicians whose problems were revealed by the Virginia licensure application. This questionnaire asks if the practitioner has ever been addicted to drugs or alcohol or has had psychiatric problems (Table 9-III). If the response is affirmative, the board's Psychiatric Advisory Committee evaluates the problem in regard to its seriousness, the degree to which it impairs professional competence, and the need for treatment. When therapy is indicated, it is provided by independent psychiatrists, who often but not always are suggested by the Psychiatry Advisory Committee. However, the board has found that most attending psychiatrists seldom report other than favorable results of treatment. Consequently, the board has had to depend on its own Psychiatric Advisory Committee to evaluate the progress toward recovery of mentally ill physicians and to determine when they can safely return to clinical practice. Continuing surveillance has enabled the Psychiatric Advisory Committee to recognize relapses at an early stage and to judge when further treatment has been sufficiently effective to again approve a return to work. It should be understood that the committee never undertakes therapy but acts solely in an advisory and evaluative capacity.

The board's experience in handling senile physicians has been limited, a total of only eight cases in ten years. However, senility has been a recognized factor in other disciplinary problems handled by the board, although it was not cited as the primary complaint. Although the number of physicians affected by a significant degree of senility who continue to practice is unknown, there are probably very few communities without at least one or more elderly physicians whose competence is a cause for concern among their colleagues (Table 9-III).

Among the more difficult cases the Virginia board has handled have been those of physicians charged with providing diagnosis and treatment not up to approved local standards. There have been fifteen such cases reported during the ten years of our study (Table 9-III). Each case required extensive investigation, frequently with formal hearings that included calling witnesses. The investigations were extremely time-consuming, and many times guilt was not proved. Such cases might better be handled at the local level where records and witnesses would be more accessible.

Reports of unprofessional conduct have also been difficult for the board to resolve. Most such cases have involved physicians who allegedly engaged in improper or inappropriate relationships with patients (Table 9-III). Disciplinary action in ten cases depended on having reliable witnesses and complainants who were willing to testify. For various reasons, witnesses often would not testify or confront the physicians involved at hearings, and many times the physician's legal counsel was able to cast significant doubt on the reliability and integrity of witnesses. Despite those impediments, a significant number of successful disciplinary actions were taken.

The reporting of physicians for fraud has been a recent phenomenon. Until 1973, this type of violation was seldom reported to the Virginia board. Most of these cases have resulted from excessively high or fradulent charges reported by Medicare or Medicaid authorities (Table 9-III).

The board has received many complaints of persons practicing medicine without a license. These cases have included imposters, cultists, and individuals with nonmedical degrees who have used their semiprofessional backgrounds to surreptitiously attempt to practice medicine (Table 9-III). Considerable investigative effort is involved in this type of case, since all aspects of the complaint must be fully documented and witnessed.

Finally, a variety of other complaints relating to infractions of the Virginia Medical Code have reached the Board. These complaints include such citations as poor records on narcotics, overcharging patients (other than outright fraud), and illegal advertising (Table 9-III).

The Virginia experience in "policing" the medical profession is relatively small in relation to the number of licensed physicians practicing in the state during the period surveyed, but we believe it is unique in its completeness (Table 9-IV). During the past ten years, the Virginia State Board of Medicine has made a strenuous effort to protect the citizens of the state from incompetent medical practitioners. As the statistics presented show, there are still many areas of weakness in the surveillance and reporting system under which the board operates. Efforts continue to strengthen and otherwise improve the program.

It is readily apparent that physicians, individually and collectively through their professional organizations, and the public must demonstrate increasing concern with all elements of professional competence if state boards are to increase their effectiveness.

REFERENCES

1. AMA News Release: Summary sheet of national medical disciplinary actions, June 19, 1977, Chicago.
2. CODE OF VIRGINIA — Chap. 12, V, Sec. 54-317(11).
3. Cahalan, D. and Cisin, I. H.: American drinking practices — summary of findings from a national probability sample. *Q J Stud Alcohol, 29*:130-151, (Mar.-June) 1968.

INDEX

A

Abortion, illegal, 58
Abuse, behavioral problem of, 53
Addict, the terminally ill, 63
Addicting drug, selection of, 28
Addiction, factors precipitating, 27
Administration Procedure Acts, 69-70
Alabama Board of Optometry, 70
Alcohol, misuse of, 28, 35, 36, 74
Alcoholics Anonymous, 38, 40, 41
Alcoholism among physicians, 35-42
Alcoholism, medical school curricula and, 37
AMA-accredited courses, 18
AMA and continuing education, 12
AMA Board of Trustees, 5
AMA Conference of Disabled Physicians, 8
AMA Council on Mental Health, 7-8
AMA House of Delegates, resolution on addiction to drugs and alcohol, 6
AMA Medical Disciplinary Committee, 5-6
AMA Physician Recognition Award Program, 13, 15
American Academy of Family Physicians, 17
American Board of Medical Specialties, 16
Attitude of public toward medical profession, 3
Authority for compliance to educational requirements, 11, 17

B

Behavioral problems among physicians, 53-64
Budd, John H., 9
Bylaws, hospital staff, 76

C

Case reports
  overbilling, 59
  senility, 55-57
  state licensing, 59
Certification, loss of, 16
CHAMPUS program, 60
Civil Rights Act of 1964, 70
Clearinghouse for major disciplinary actions, 6
Commitment to state or private hospitals, 38
Competence, maintaining professional, 11-19
Conduct, unprofessional, 53
Consumerism and medical profession, 5
Continuing education
  for competence, 12, 13, 17
  New Mexico bill requiring, 7
Currency of professional skills, problems of maintaining, 13

D

Definition, alcohol abuse, 35
Delegation of physician responsibility, problem of, 59
Demand for professional discipline, 3-10
Depression
  and drug-addicted physician, 22
  in physicians, cause of illness, 48-49
  problem of recognizing, 75-76
Derbyshire, Robert C., 7, 13
Deterants to maintaining competence, 14
Deviant behavior, problem of recognition of, 75-76
Disabled doctors, AMA conference on, 8
Disciplinary actions by Medical Boards, 82
Disciplinary procedure, Board hearings

97